Text Atlas of Pathology of the Foot

Text Atlas of Pathology of the Foot

Ruggero Caputo MD
Professor and Chairman
Istituto di scienze dermatologiche
Ospedale maggiore
Policlinico IRCCS
Università degli studi di Milano
Milan, Italy

Stefano Veraldi MD
Senior Researcher
Istituto di scienze dermatologiche
Ospedale maggiore
Policlinico IRCCS
Università degli studi di Milano
Milan, Italy

Federico Annoni MD
Associate Professor
Istituto di chirurgia generale
e oncologia chirurgica
Ospedale maggiore
Policlinico IRCCS
Università degli studi di Milano
Milan, Italy

MARTIN DUNITZ

© Martin Dunitz Ltd 2000

First published in the United Kingdom in 2000 by
Martin Dunitz Ltd
The Livery House
7–9 Pratt Street
London NW1 0AE
Tel: +44-(0)20-7482-2202
Fax: +44-(0)20-7267-0159
E-mail: info@mdunitz.globalnet.co.uk
Web site: http://www.dunitz.co.uk

A CIP catalogue record for this title is available
from the British Library.

ISBN 1–85317–787–3

Distributed in the United States by:
Blackwell Science Inc.
Commerce Place, 350 Main Street
Malden MA 02148, USA
Tel: 1-800-215-1000

Distributed in Canada by:
Login Brothers Book Company
324 Salteaux Crescent
Winnipeg, Manitoba R3J 3T2
Canada
Tel: 204-224-4068

Distributed in Brazil by:
Ernesto Reichmann Distribuidora de Livros, Ltda
Rua Coronel Marques 335, Tatuape 03440-000
São Paulo
Brazil

Composition by Scribe Design, Gillingham, Kent
Printed and bound in Italy by Printer Trento Srl

Contents

5   Miscellaneous disorders   169

Preface

Skin lesions of the feet are, today, more and more frequently brought to the attention of dermatologists. This appears not only to be a consequence of patients suffering from troublesome foot disorders but also as a consequence of changes in lifestyles. Requests to dermatologists come from colleagues involved in such areas as orthopaedics and sport medicine who wish to obtain a correct diagnosis for disorders that have often been misinterpreted, underestimated or ill-treated.

This atlas has been produced with the intention of providing dermatologists with easily comparable images of the various skin disorders that are either specific to the feet, that have manifested themselves in an unusual location or that are localized manifestations of a more diffuse dermatosis. The authors have classed as foot disorders skin lesions that involve the areas below the ankles. Nail disorders have not been included since these have already been well described elsewhere. Dermatological disorders of the feet have been divided into four main groups: inflammatory diseases, proliferative diseases, hereditary and keratinization disorders, and infectious and parasitic diseases. The chapter entitled 'Miscellaneous disorders' gathers together all the conditions that do not fall into any of these four groupings. In an attempt to make comparison easier, in each chapter disorders characterized by similar clinical features have been grouped together. For each disorder, a brief definition is provided, the site-related features of the diseases are illustrated (when, of course, the disorder is not specific to the feet), and a differential diagnosis is made, mainly on the basis of clinical criteria.

It is hoped this atlas will be a handy, easy-to-use tool for the dermatologist as well as for all other physicians who have to deal with 'feet problems'.

Ruggero Caputo
Stefano Veraldi
Federico Annoni

Acknowledgements

The majority of the illustrations in this book come from the collection of the Institute of Dermatological Science of the University of Milan. However, a few have been provided by the following colleagues: Elvio Alessi, Nicola Aste, Claudine Blanchet-Bardon, Vera Dal Pozzo, Aldo Finzi, Carlo Gelmetti and Antonella Tosti. They are acknowledged in the legends to the figures.

1 Inflammatory diseases

ATOPIC DERMATITIS
JUVENILE PLANTAR DERMATOSIS
POMPHOLYX (dyshidrotic eczema)
CONTACT DERMATITIS
PHYTODERMATITIS AND PHYTOPHOTODERMATITIS
PSORIASIS
INFANTILE ACROPUSTULOSIS
LICHEN PLANUS
LICHEN STRIATUS
PITYRIASIS LICHENOIDES
GRANULOMA ANNULARE
ERYTHEMA MULTIFORME
DERMATITIS HERPETIFORMIS
LINEAR IgA DERMATOSIS OF CHILDHOOD
EPIDERMOLYSIS BULLOSA ACQUISITA
ERYTHEMA ELEVATUM DIUTINUM
PYODERMA GANGRENOSUM
SYSTEMIC LUPUS ERYTHEMATOSUS
CAPILLARITIS OF THE INFERIOR LIMBS
HENOCH–SCHÖNLEIN PURPURA OR ANAPHYLACTOID PURPURA
DYSPROTEINAEMIC PURPURA
DRUG-INDUCED PURPURA
LOCALIZED SCLERODERMA
LICHEN SCLEROSUS ET ATROPHICUS

ATOPIC DERMATITIS

Atopic dermatitis is a chronic, fluctuating disease characterized by three major symptoms: atopy, pruritus and eczema. The age of onset is usually 2–6 months following birth. The cutaneous lesions are polymorphic (erythema, vesicles, papules, scaling, crusting) and recurrent. These lesions tend to merge into plaques that have ill-defined borders and that involve the face, the anticubital and popliteal fossae, the wrists and the lateral aspects of the legs in a symmetrical fashion. Juvenile plantar dermatosis is a specific form of atopic dermatitis.

Clinical features

The type of skin lesion depends on the disease's phase of evolution. The feet may be involved at any age, but most commonly in childhood or adult forms. This involvement consists of papular or lichenified plaques. The sites most commonly affected are the ankles and the dorsal aspect of the feet and toes. The soles are frequently dry and scaly.

Differential diagnosis

In allergic contact dermatitis the patch tests are positive.

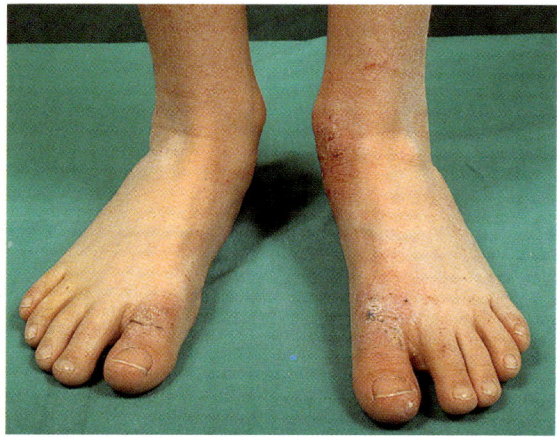

Figure 1.1
Atopic dermatitis. In this adolescent patient the lesions are lichenified; they involve the ankles and the dorsal aspect of the feet and of the first toe symmetrically.

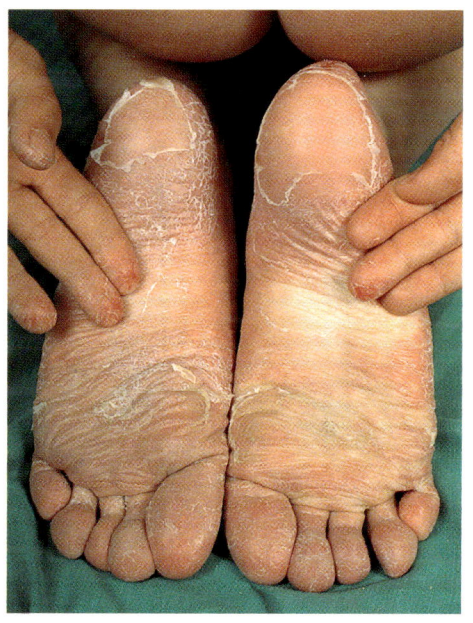

Figure 1.2
Atopic dermatitis. The skin of the soles is frequently dry and scaling. In this child, similar lesions are also present on the palms.

JUVENILE PLANTAR DERMATOSIS

Juvenile plantar dermatosis is a chronic condition (most probably related to an atopy) that is characterized by dry, red, fissured skin symmetrically involving the plantar surface of the toes and the anterior third of the sole. The skin has a glazed and cracked appearance.

The interdigital spaces are spared. Pruritus is absent. The condition occurs almost exclusively in children under the age of 15 years.

Differential diagnosis

Contact dermatitis is differentiated by the absence of pruritus and vesicles and by negative patch tests.

Psoriasis presents with a scalloped and erythematous margin.

Tinea pedis frequently involves the interdigital spaces and both microscopical examination and culture are positive.

Pompholyx is characterized by deep-seated vesicles, mainly on the sides of the soles.

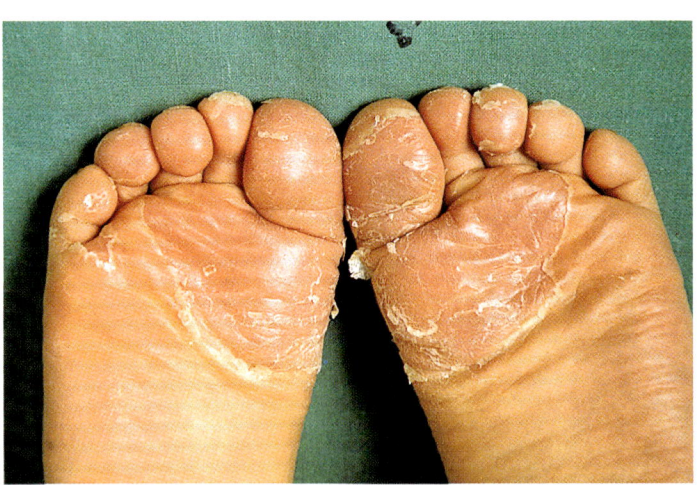

Figure 1.3

Juvenile plantar dermatosis. This term refers to scales that appear on the shiny skin of the soles of the feet in children who are atopic. The lesions involve the anterior third of the soles and the plantar surface of the toes symmetrically.

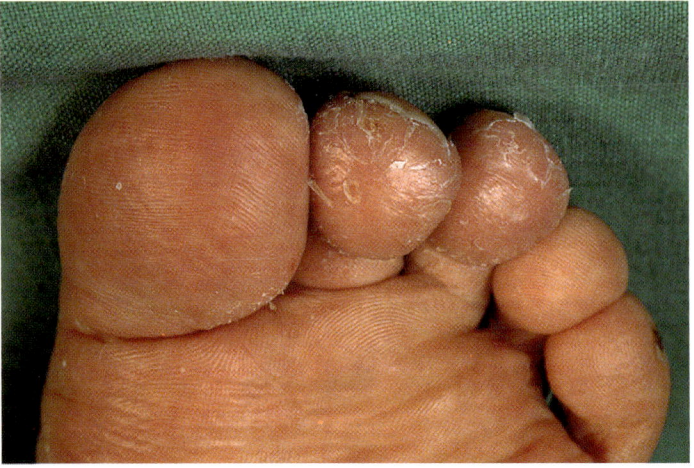

Figure 1.4

Juvenile plantar dermatosis. The skin of the plantar surface of the toes assumes a glazed and cracked appearance. Pruritus is absent.

POMPHOLYX (dyshidrotic eczema)

Dyshidrotic eczema or pompholyx is a spongiotic dermatitis of the palms and soles. It is characterized by recurrent eruptions of deep-seated vesicles that are usually distributed symmetrically. Itching is sporadic and may precede the eruption of vesicles. Resolution with desquamation occurs in 2–3 weeks. The disease is more common before the age of 40 years.

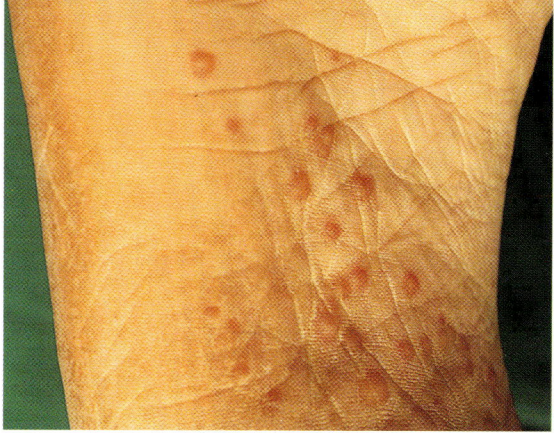

Figure 1.5
Dyshidrosis. Deep-seated vesicles localized on the soles of the feet are the typical early lesions of the disease.

Clinical features

There is a sudden onset of crops of vesicles that resemble tapioca on the soles or along the sides of the toes. Blisters may develop in the same localization.

Differential diagnosis

Tinea pedis may be vesicular but it is usually located unilaterally. Microscopical examination demonstrates hyphae.

Contact dermatitis may be excluded by patch testing.

In pustular psoriasis the primary lesions are sterile pustules within areas of erythema.

Hand-foot-and-mouth disease is characterized by discrete, oblong-shaped vesicles and by the involvement of the oral mucosa. It typically affects young children.

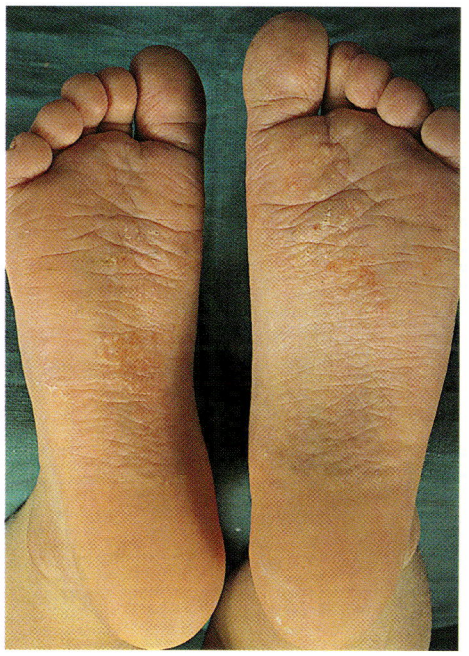

Figure 1.6
Dyshidrosis. Tense vesicles coalesce and assume the appearance of tapioca. The lesions are frequently distributed symmetrically.

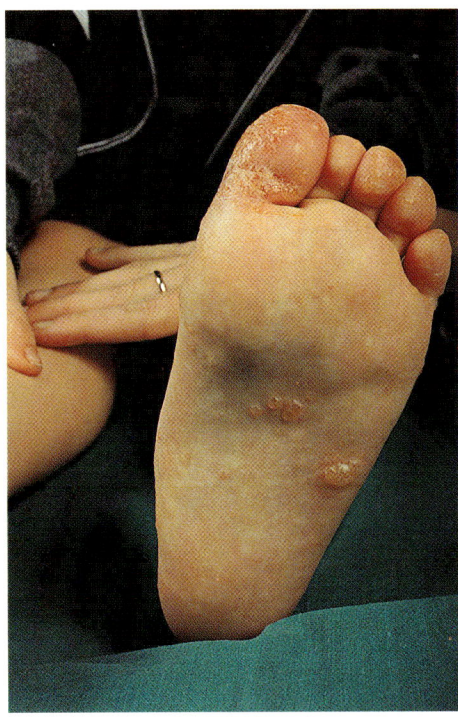

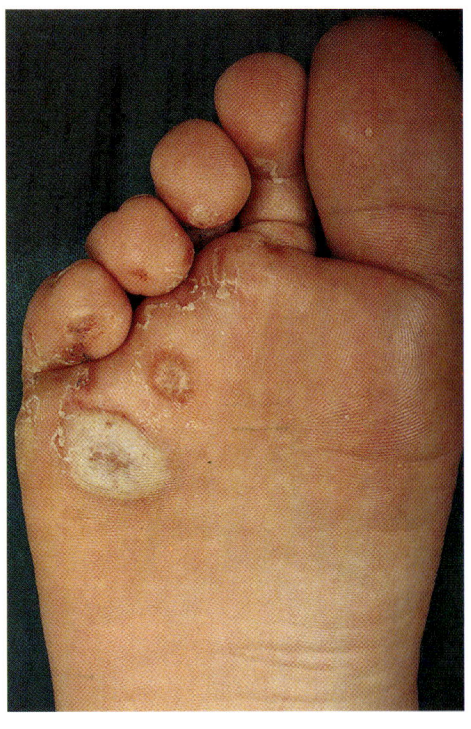

Figure 1.7

Dyshidrosis. Large bullae may occasionally be noted.

Figure 1.8

Dyshidrosis. Resolution occurs with desquamation in 2–3 weeks. Scale crusts may involve the sides of the toes. During their development, as in this example, the bullae may assume annular or target-like shapes.

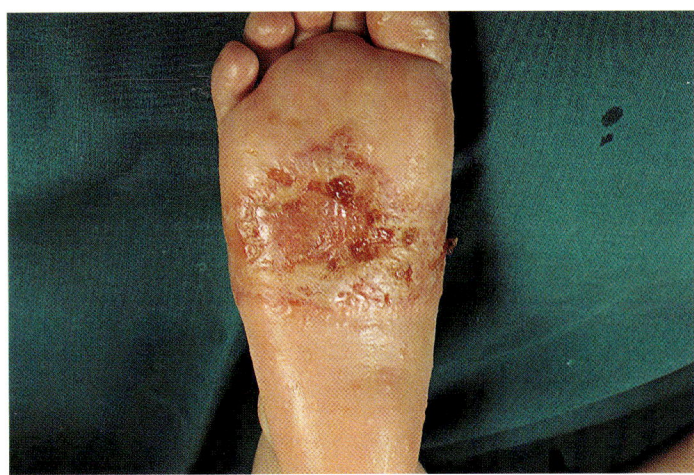

Figure 1.9

Dyshidrosis. In this patient, the inflammatory pustular bullous lesions are a consequence of impetiginization.

CONTACT DERMATITIS

Contact dermatitis is an inflammatory reaction that follows immediately after direct contact with an irritant (irritant contact dermatitis) or within several days of direct contact with an allergen (allergic contact dermatitis). As in atopic dermatitis, the cutaneous lesions of allergic contact dermatitis are polymorphic (erythema, vesicles, papules, scaling, crusting) and these are accompanied by intense itching. The lesions are (at least initially) localized to the area that came into contact with the irritant or allergens. Irritant contact dermatitis occurs quickly, and the lesions bypass the papular stage, proceeding directly from redness to blisters.

Clinical features

Shoes are mainly responsible for allergic contact dermatitis on the feet. Shoe dermatitis presents as erythema and then scaling of the dorsal aspect of the feet. The soles are rarely affected because of the protection afforded by the thick stratum corneum. The most frequent causative allergens are potassium dichromate, nickel sulphate, glutaraldeide, thiuram x, 2-mercapto-benzothiazole and dibutylthiourea.

Patch tests are necessary for a correct diagnosis.

Differential diagnosis

Tinea pedis involves the webs between the toes and the soles much more commonly than the dorsal aspect of the feet.

Psoriasis involves the soles more than the dorsa and is often associated with pits in the nail plates.

Dyshidrotic dermatitis may be indistinguishable from allergic contact dermatitis; however, the vesicles tend more frequently to be aligned along the sides of toes.

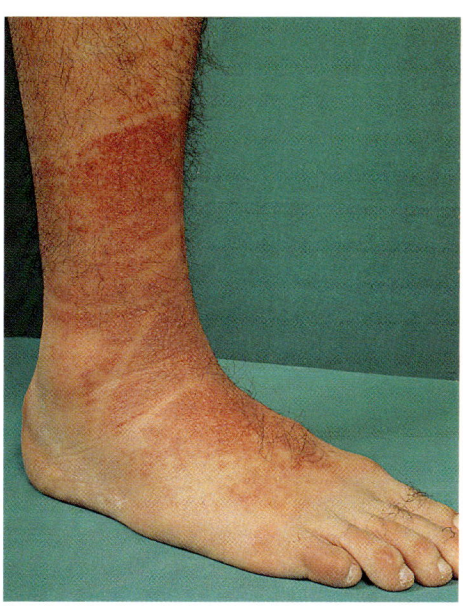

Figure 1.10
Irritant contact dermatitis. These erythematous lesions are the consequence of a skin irritation caused by an occlusive bandage.

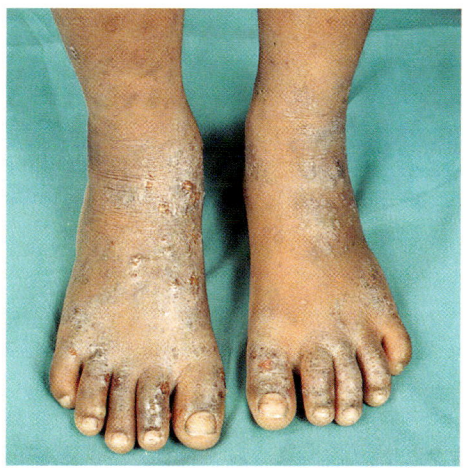

Figure 1.11
Allergic contact dermatitis. Polymorphic lesions (erythema, vesicles, scales and crusts) in a patient who has become sensitized to potassium dichromate and nickel sulphate.

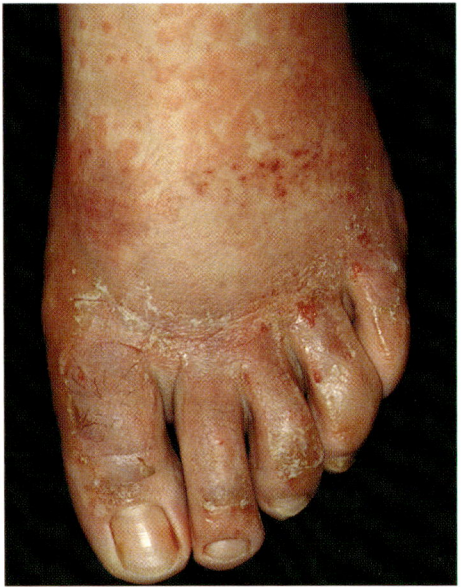

Figure 1.12
Allergic contact dermatitis. In this example, papules covered by scales have appeared on the dorsum of the feet and the toes as a result of sensitization to paraphenylendiamine.

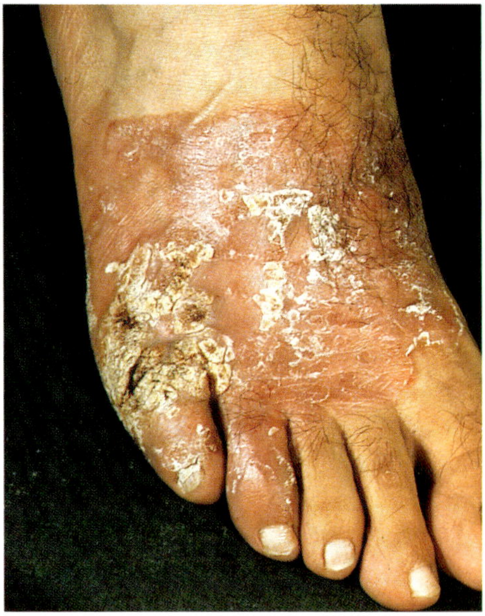

Figure 1.13
Allergic contact dermatitis. This large erythematous-scaly patch has appeared as a result of sensitization to neomycin that was applied topically.

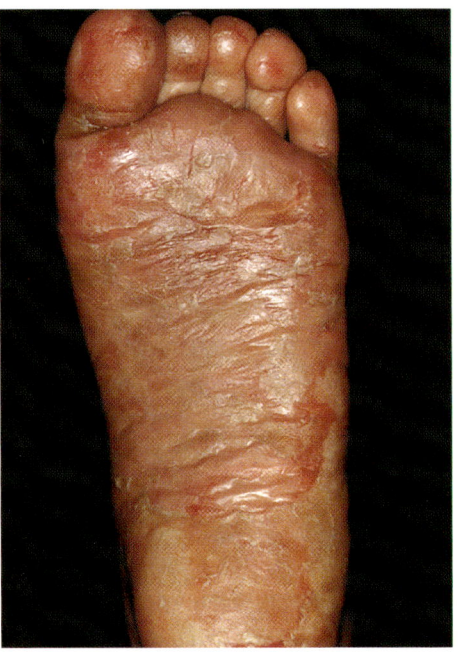

Figure 1.14
Allergic contact dermatitis. This erythematous-scaly lesion, which involves the whole sole, is the consequence of an allergic reaction to an antiperspirant.

PHYTODERMATITIS AND PHYTOPHOTODERMATITIS

Phytodermatitis is an acute inflammatory reaction caused by the skin coming into contact with certain plants. The pathogenic mechanism may be toxic, irritative or allergic.

If the contact is followed by exposure to sunlight, phytophotodermatitis will be induced. In such cases, the pathogenic mechanism may again be toxic, irritative or allergic.

All races, both sexes and people of any age may be affected. In temperate climates these disorders are more frequent during the summer, while they will occur all the year round in tropical and subtropical areas.

The limbs are the most frequently involved sites.

Clinical features

The eruption is typically erythematous, vesicular and bullous, with a strange shape, distribution and arrangement. The type of eruption also depends on the species of plant involved and how the contact was made. The blisters may be very large, filled with serous fluid and are often not surrounded by an erythematous halo. Burning and pruritus are always present and often severe. A postinflammatory brown hyperpigmentation often persists for months.

Differential diagnosis

The clinical history of the disorder must be carefully taken, as the patient will usually provide the diagnosis.

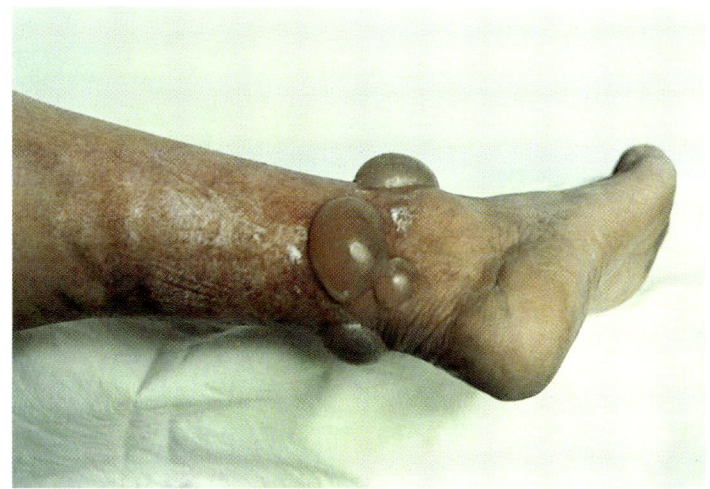

Figure 1.15
Phytodermatitis. Very large blisters with serous fluid.

PSORIASIS

Psoriasis is one of the most common chronic skin diseases, affecting some 1.5–2% of the population. It is characterized by sharply demarcated, erythematous scaling lesions that especially involve the scalp and the extensor surfaces. Many clinical forms may occur, and pustules may be present. Broadly speaking, symptoms can be grouped as evidence of either 'psoriasis vulgaris' or 'pustular psoriasis'. One third of patients develop the disease before the age of 20 years. Histologically, the main findings are parakeratosis, a decrease in the thickness of the granular zone and spongiform pustules that are full of neutrophils.

Clinical features

Psoriasis vulgaris causes sharply demarcated, red, scaly lesions to extend on the lateral surface of the feet. The well defined edges and erythematous borders of the lesions are important features for diagnosis. The heels frequently demonstrate marked hyperkeratosis with deep rhagades.

Pustular psoriasis is characterized by recurrent crops of sterile pustules, 2–4 mm in diameter within the areas of erythema. These lesions may remain isolated or may merge into erythematous, scaly plaques where pustules at all stages of development are observed. The lateral border of the foot, the instep and the sides or back of the heel are the sites of infection. The whole sole is less frequently involved.

The so-called acrodermatitis continua of Hallopeau initially affects the tip of a toe, with erythema, pustules and scaling. The lesions extend progressively and may be bordered by a fringe of undermined epidermis. The nail-plate may be completely destroyed.

Differential diagnosis

Psoriasis vulgaris

- Hyperkeratotic eczema: less sharply defined lesions, the presence of vesicles and itching.
- Tinea pedis: direct microscopic examination and culture are necessary for diagnosis.
- Pityriasis rubra pilaris: characterized by the salmon colour of the soles. Follicular keratoic papules on the dorsal aspect of the feet.
- Hereditary palmoplantar keratodermas: less sharply defined lesions, absence of erythematous scaly edges and the presence of associated anomalies.
- Lichen planus: at the periphery of the lesions, shiny, flat-topped lichenoid papules.
- Paraneoplastic acrokeratosis (Bazex's syndrome): cutaneous changes develop gradually, also involving the hands, ears and nose.
- Secondary syphilis: characterized by its copper-coloured, peripherical scaling papules, positive serology and dark-field examination.

Pustular psoriasis

- Contact dermatitis: itching and vesicular involvement, mainly of the dorsal aspect of the feet.
- Dyshidrotic eczema: deep-seated vesicles or pustules mainly located on the sides of soles; recurrent attacks with spontaneous remissions.
- Tinea pedis: unilaterally located; positive microscopic examination and culture.

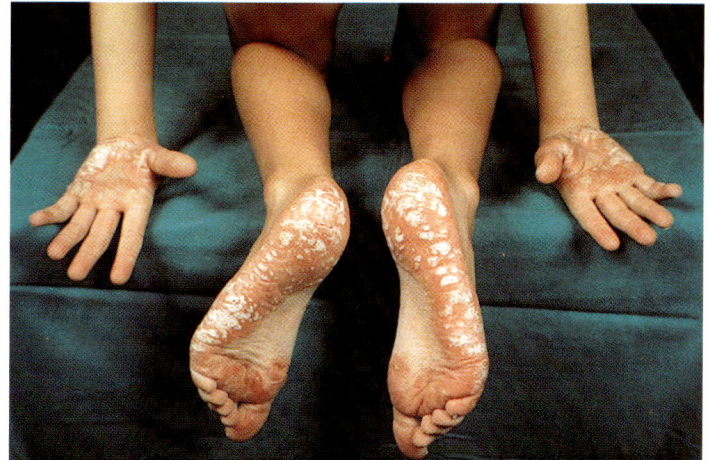

Figure 1.16
Psoriasis vulgaris. These typical erythematous scaly lesions are located symmetrically on the palms and soles

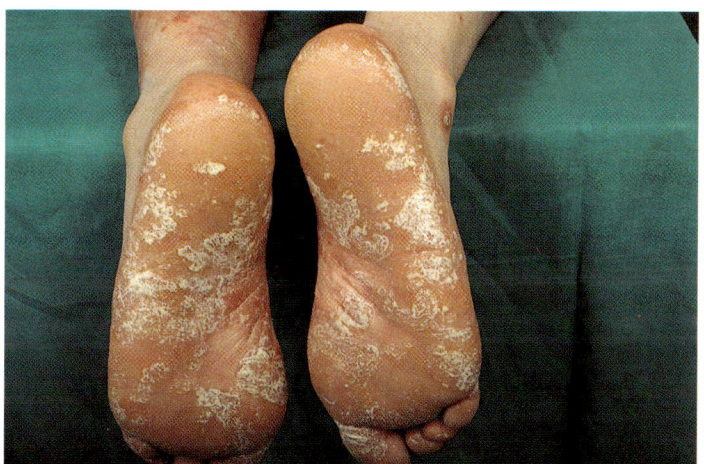

Figure 1.17
Psoriasis vulgaris. Scaling is particularly apparent on the soles of this patient.

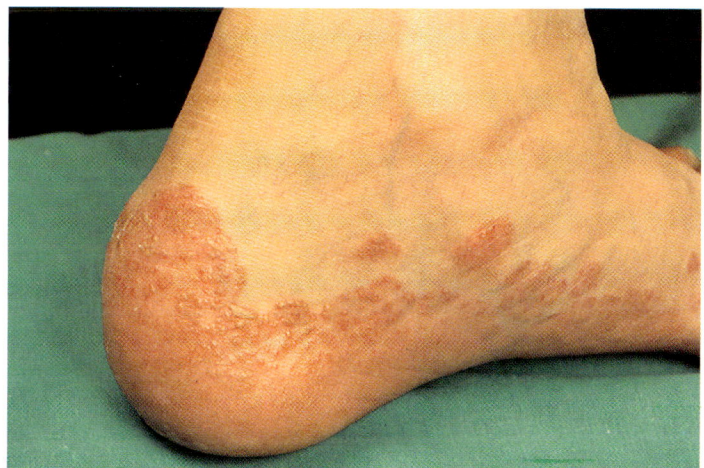

Figure 1.18
Psoriasis vulgaris. Well defined edges are an important criterion in the diagnosis of this complaint. The heel is also frequently involved.

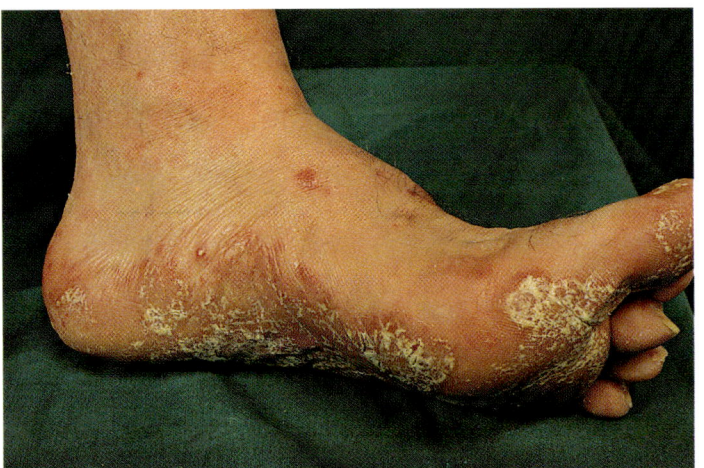

Figure 1.19

Psoriasis vulgaris. The sharply demarcated, red, scaly lesions often extend to the lateral surface of the foot. Note also the presence of an isolated pustule.

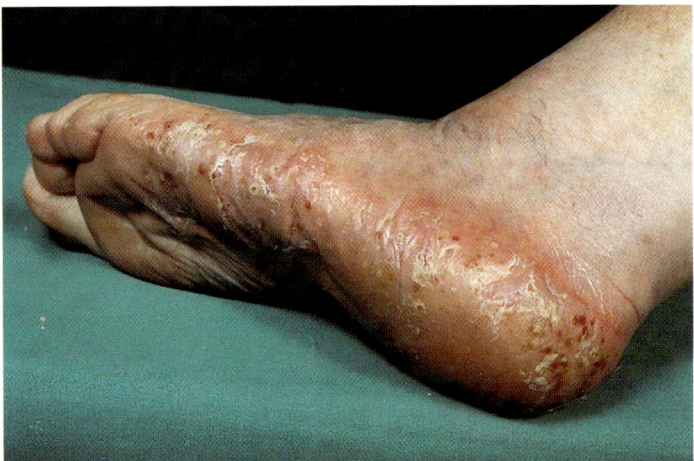

Figure 1.20

Pustular psoriasis. Lesions in this condition are sterile pustules 2–4 mm in diameter located within areas of erythema. The disease may be restricted to the palms and soles (Barber's variety).

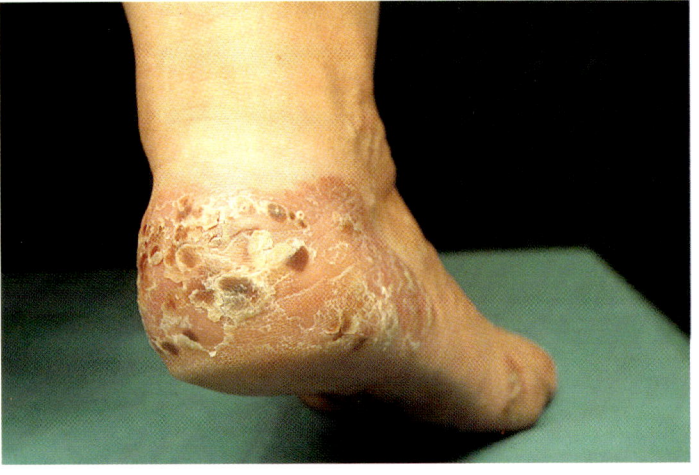

Figure 1.21

Pustular psoriasis. In this patient pustules at all stages of development are present on the back of the heel – which is a common site of infection.

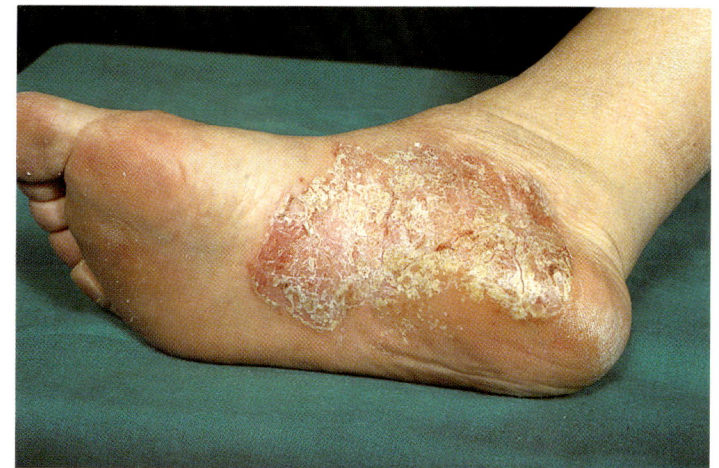

Figure 1.22

Pustular psoriasis. In this patient there is a well demarcated patch of pustular psoriasis on the lateral border of the foot. Note that the lesion is bordered with a fringe of undermined epidermis.

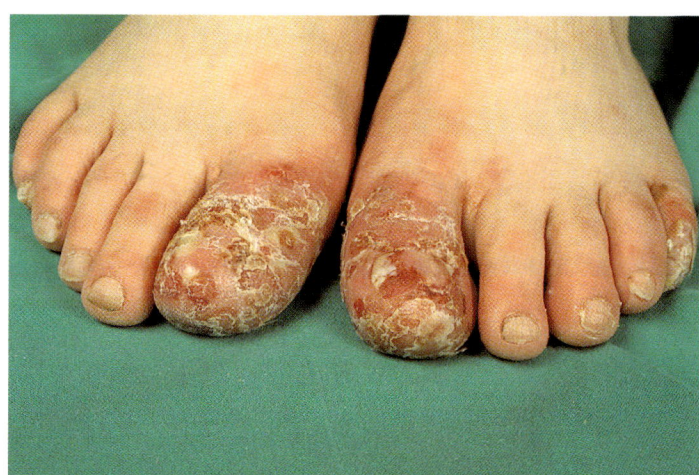

Figure 1.23

Acrodermatitis continua of Hallopeau. This particular form of pustular psoriasis affects, at least in the early stages, the tip of the toes. Erythema, pustules and scaling are present. The lesions extend progressively, ultimately destroying the nail-plate completely.

INFANTILE ACROPUSTULOSIS

Infantile acropustulosis is a rare disease of unknown aetiology that is most common in black children. It is characterized by crops of eruptive, pruritic, vesicular pustules that involve the distal extremities. Onset is generally between the first and tenth months following birth. Spontaneous resolution occurs before the age of 4 years. Eosinophilia is present. Histologically the pustules are unilocular and intradermal containing neutrophils and eosinophils in varying amounts.

Clinical features

The onset of pruritic vesicles or pustules is rapid (within 24 hours). The plantar area is more often involved than the dorsal surface of the foot. The lesions are recurrent and resistant to treatment.

Differential diagnosis

Scabies is differentiated by the presence of mites and eggs, which can be demonstrated by scraping.

Transient neonatal pustular melanosis is present at birth. It resolves spontaneously in 3 months and normally affects the trunk.

Pustular psoriasis is rare in early infancy. It is characterized by recurrent crops of pustules within areas of erythema and scaling.

In candidiasis, periodic acid-Schiff (PAS) stain demonstrates hyphae or pseudohyphae not only in the horny layer but also within the pustules themselves.

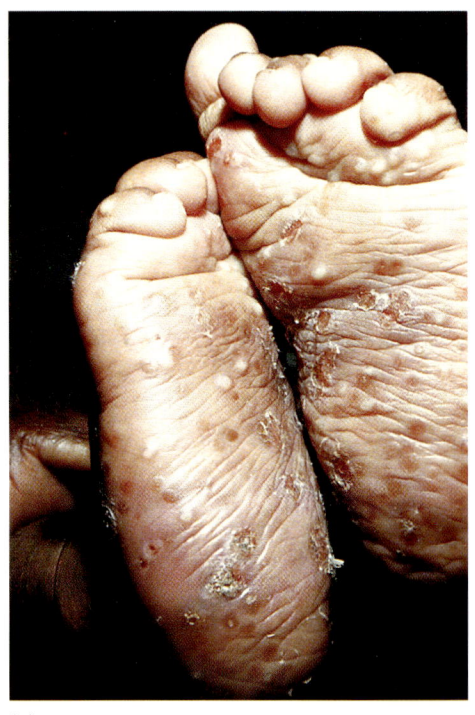

(a)

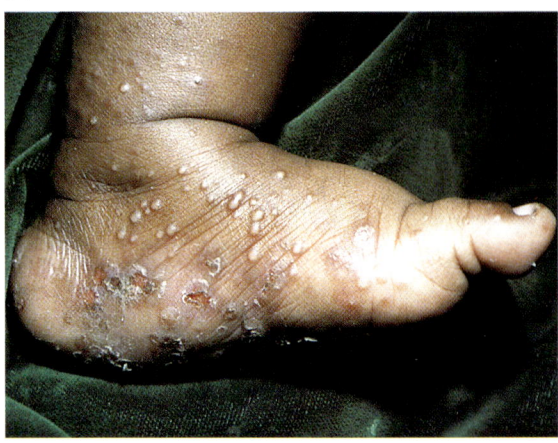

(b)

Figure 1.24(a,b)

Infantile acropustolosis. Eruptive, pruritic vesicular pustules can be observed on the feet of this black infant. The lesions are recurrent and resistant to treatment. Eosinophilia is a common finding.

LICHEN PLANUS

Lichen planus (LP) is a common, pruritic, chronic papular mucocutaneous disease that mainly affects patients in the third to sixth decade of life. LP may exhibit numerous variations in pattern, with differences in the morphology and configuration of the lesions. The classic form is characterized by violaceous, shiny, flat-topped, scaly, polygonal papules typically located on the flexor aspects of the wrist and forearms, the extensor aspects of the hand and ankles, and the lumbar region. The soles are rarely affected. Pigmentary sequelae are frequently observed, but these are temporary. Histologically, the papule consists of a sub-epidermal, band-like lymphocytic infiltrate that is associated with the destruction of the basal cell layer, hypergranulosis and hyperkeratosis.

Clinical features

Classic, hypertrophic bullous and ulcerative patterns are seen on the dorsal aspect of the feet. The hypertrophic pattern is characterized by firm, reddish-brown, violaceous, verrucous plaques. The bullous pattern consists of vesiculobullous lesions associated with patches of classic LP. Ulcerative LP of the feet is painful and may be associated with the permanent loss of the toenails and with cicatricial alopecia. On the soles, lesions may be papular and warty or, more rarely, bullous and ulcerative.

Differential diagnosis

The typical LP lesions on the dorsal aspects of the feet must be differentiated from lichenoid eruption induced by drugs such as antihypertensive, antimalarial and antiinflammatory drugs and from graph-versus-host disease.

Hypertrophic lesions may be confused by localized neurodermatitis and histopathology may be necessary for a correct diagnosis.

Papular, hyperkeratotic lesions of the soles must be differentiated from psoriasis (characterized by the presence of other typical lesions, scalloped margins and the absence of itching), secondary syphilis (copper-coloured, peripherical, scaly papules, positive serology and dark-field examination) and warts (characterized by reddish brown dots). In the absence of concurrent characteristic papular lesions, ulcerative LP of the soles always needs a histopathological examination.

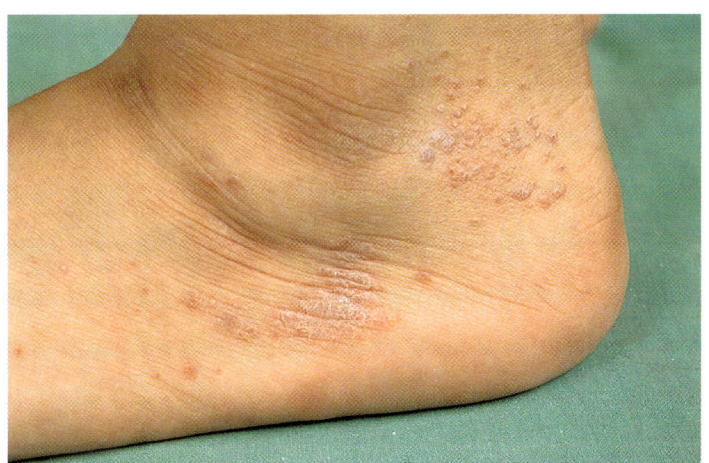

Figure 1.25
Classic lichen ruber planus. The lesions consist of violaceous, shiny, flat-topped, polygonal pruritic papules.

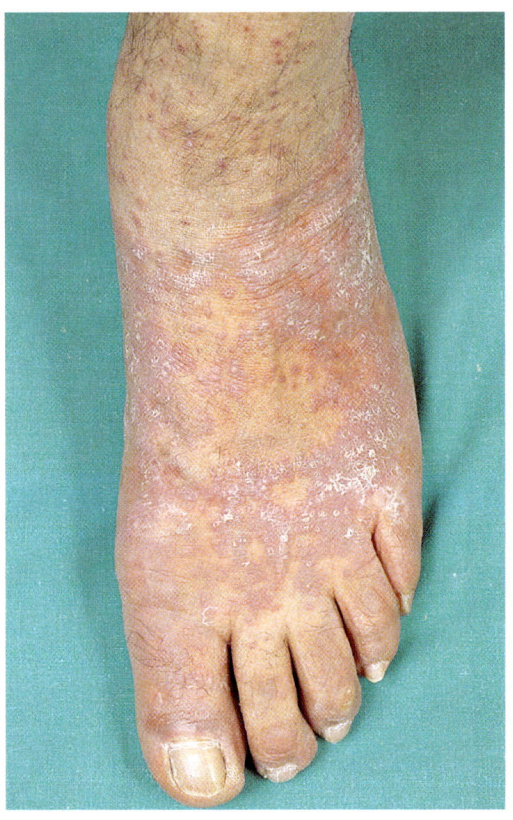

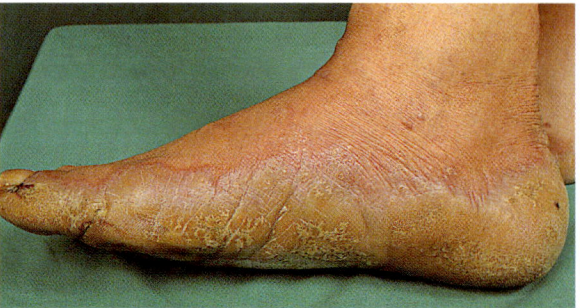

Figure 1.27

Classic lichen ruber planus. On the soles, the lesions become hyperkeratotic, with deep rhagades. Note the violaceous border and the small quantity of shiny papules that are typical of this condition. These are located on the back of the foot.

Figure 1.26

Classic lichen ruber planus. In this condition the papules may merge to form violaceous, scaly plaques. The whitish, lacy, reticulated pattern in this example is typical of lichen planus (Wickham's striae).

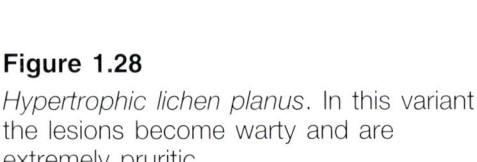

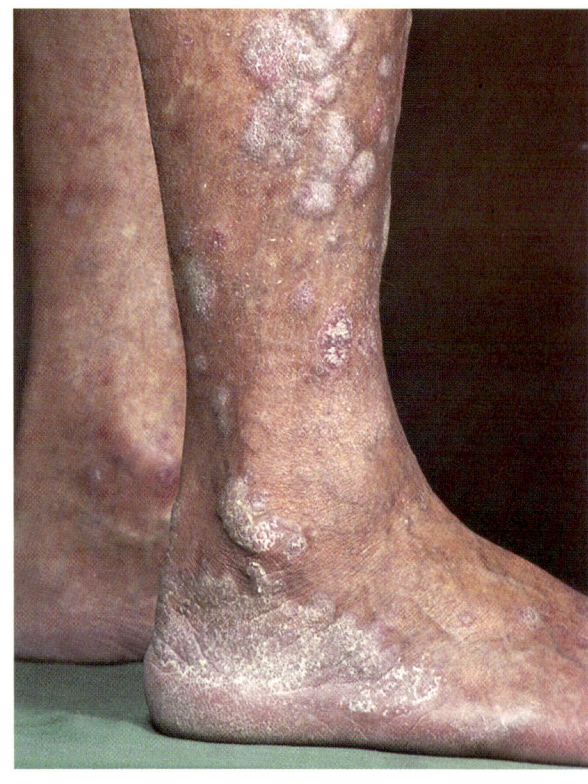

Figure 1.28

Hypertrophic lichen planus. In this variant the lesions become warty and are extremely pruritic.

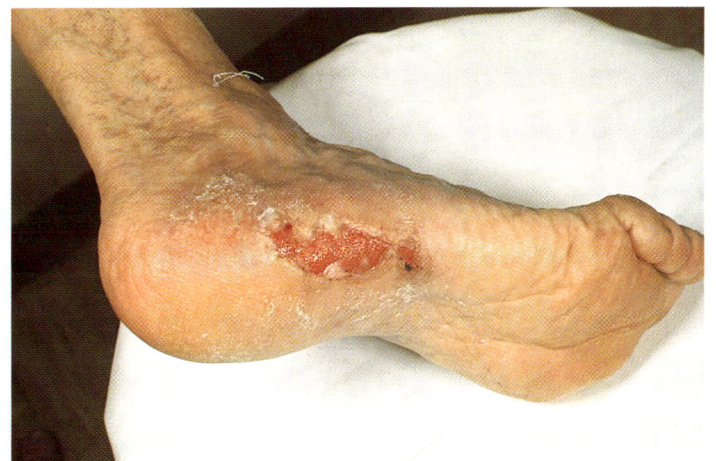

Figure 1.29

Bullous lichen planus. Located on the sole, these lesions rapidly become ulcerative and are also painful.

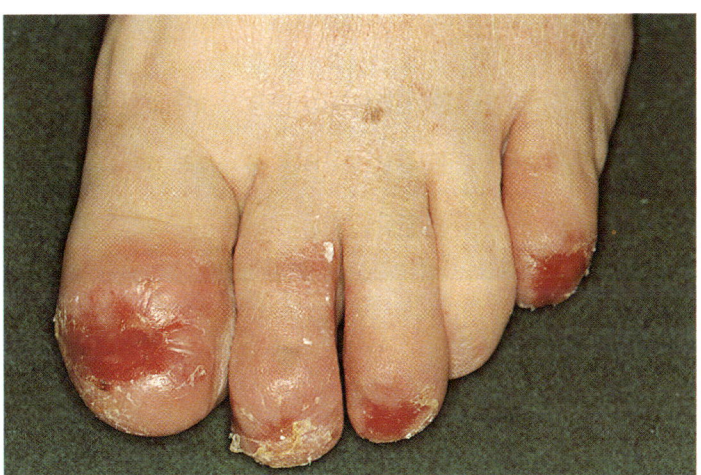

Figure 1.30

Bullous lichen planus. The permanent loss of the nails is a possible complication of this variant. (Photograph courtesy of Professor Aldo Finzi.)

LICHEN STRIATUS

Lichen striatus is the most common of the Blaschko, linearly acquired, self-limited inflammatory skin eruptions. It consists of grouped papules in linear array that form a band on one side of the body. In two thirds of cases the lesions are predominantly distributed on the limbs (47% upper limbs and 20% lower limbs). The disease is more frequent in children (the median age is 4 years). The main histological findings are focal parakeratosis, focal spongiosis, necrotic keratinocytes, infiltrate of lymphocytes at the dermo-epidermal junction, and both superficial and deep perivascular infiltrate of lymphocytes and histiocytes.

Clinical features

The elementary lesions are round, smooth or slightly verrucous papules that vary in colour from pearly white to dark red. These papules are clustered into a single, unilateral band and are a few millimetres to a few centimetres in width. This band may reach the tip of one or two digits, causing onychodystrophy. Pruritus is usually absent.

The disease resolves spontaneously in a few months (mean duration 10 months) but nail-plate involvement may persist for several years.

Differential diagnosis

*   Linear verrucous naevus is a persistent hyperkeratotic band that is present at birth.
*   Inflammatory linear verrucous naevus is an inflammatory pruritic band.
*   Linear porokeratosis consists of an atrophic band with its typical thread-like keratotic rim.

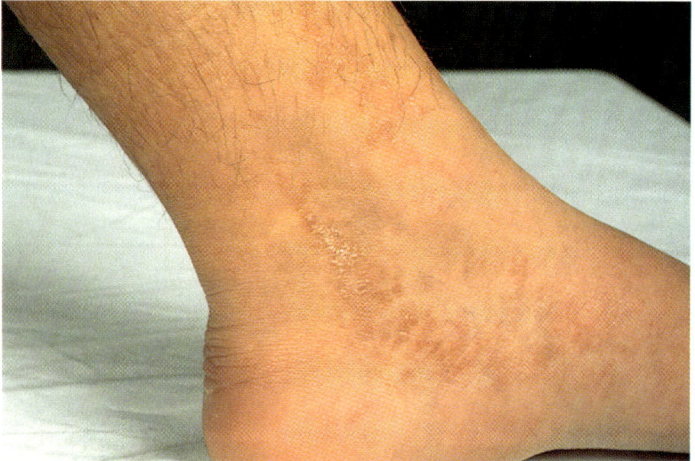

Figure 1.31
Lichen striatus. Pink, slightly hyperkeratotic papules in a somewhat linear arrangement on the lateral border of the foot are a common finding in this condition.

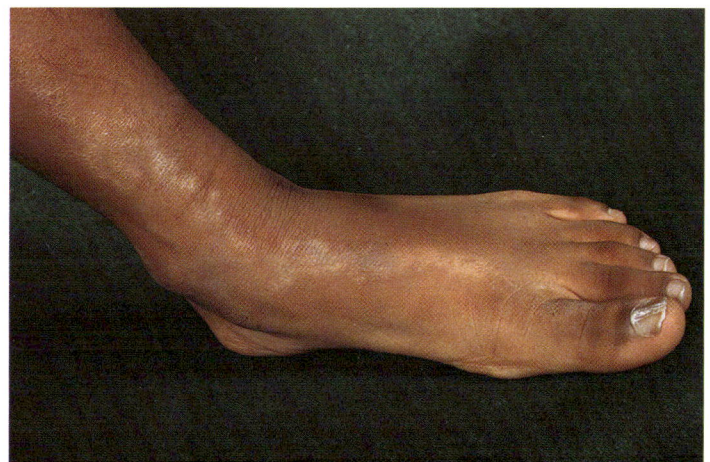

Figure 1.32

Lichen striatus. In this black patient, the band consists of whitish, slightly scaly papules and these clearly follow the Blanschko lines. Nail-plate involvement is evident.

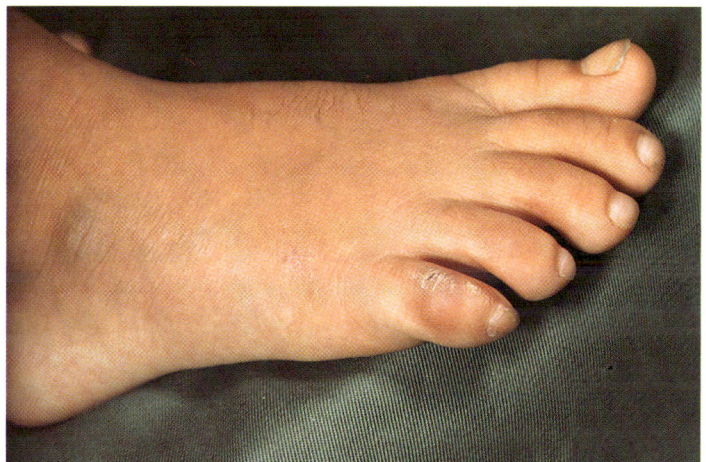

Figure 1.33

Lichen striatus. The lesion consists of a short band on the back of the fifth toe. It involves the nail-plate and has caused onychodystrophy.

PITYRIASIS LICHENOIDES

Pityriasis lichenoides (PL) – sometimes previously referred to as guttate parapsoriasis – is a self-limiting skin disorder that can affect both children and adults. It is characterized by erythematous papules that tend to evolve into scales, vesicles, pustules and crusts, sometimes with central necrosis. The disease is sub-divided into an acute form and a chronic form. The acute form consists of crops of round, reddish papules that evolve into vesicular and necrotic lesions. In the chronic form the lesions are reddish brown papules with an adherent central scale that tends to separate spontaneously. On the basis of the lesions' distribution PL may be classified as diffuse, central (localized to the trunk) and peripheral (limited to the limbs and buttocks).

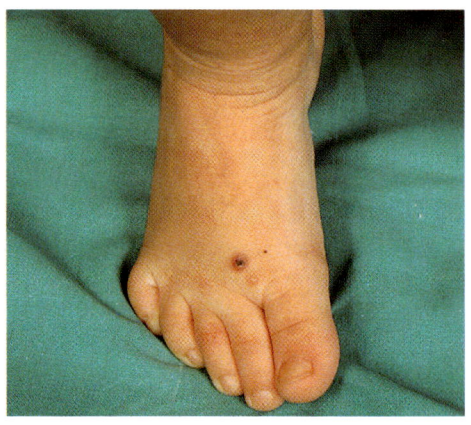

Figure 1.34
Pityriasis lichenoides. In this peripheral form a small quantity of papular scaly and papular crusted lesion is present on the dorsal aspect of the foot.

Clinical features

Polymorphous lesions are confined to the dorsal aspect of the feet in the diffuse and peripheral forms of the disease. The soles are always spared.

Differential diagnosis

In psoriasis the underlying erythema is bright, and the entire lesion is covered with white scales. In Gianotti–Crosti syndrome the papular rash associated with the disease usually lasts 15–30 days, haemorrhagic crusts are not seen. Henoch–Schönlein purpura is characterized by petechiae which may be accompanied by systemic symptoms (mainly joint and kidney involvement). In secondary syphilis the papular scaling lesions that have the typical collarette are mainly localized on the palms and soles that, in PL, are spared. Serological tests are positive.

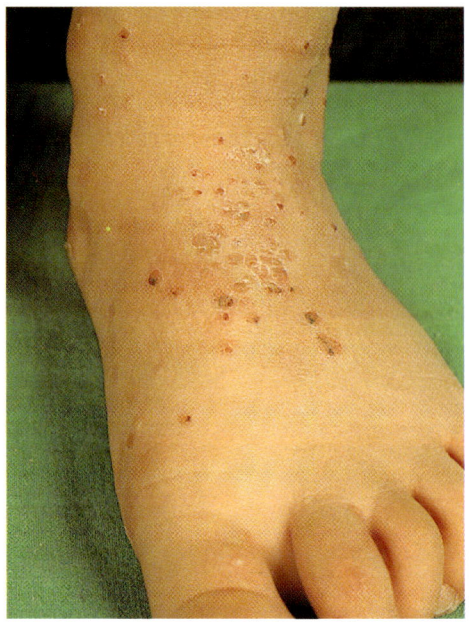

Figure 1.35
Pityriasis lichenoides. In this diffuse variant of the disease, the polymorphic nature of the lesions is apparent. Several smooth, scaly, crusted papules have invaded the back of the foot.

GRANULOMA ANNULARE

Granuloma annulare is a common, self-limiting inflammatory disease characterized by asymptomatic papules arranged in an annular fashion. In the localized form of the disease (which is the most common) the lesions involve the distal part of the upper and lower extremities.

Atypical forms (such as generalized and inflammatory forms and subcutaneous and perforating forms) are less frequent. Children and young adults are predominantly affected. The disease disappears spontaneously in 80% of patients in approximately two years, but recurrences are common. The histological aspect of the disease is characterized by histiocytes that are arranged in a palisaded manner around the necrobiotic foci of connective tissue.

Clinical features

The rings of smooth, skin-coloured, firm papules are mainly located on the dorsal surfaces of the feet. The lesions tend to enlarge centrifugally and are usually non-pruritic.

Differential diagnosis

Lesions of tinea corporis and erythema annulare centrifugum are covered by scales; in tinea corporis, both microscopical examination for fungi and cultures are positive.

Erythema multiforme consists of papules that become vesicular in shape. Annular lichen planus differs in that the colour of the papules is violaceous and the lesions are pruritic.

Annular sarcoidis may be differentiated only histopathologically.

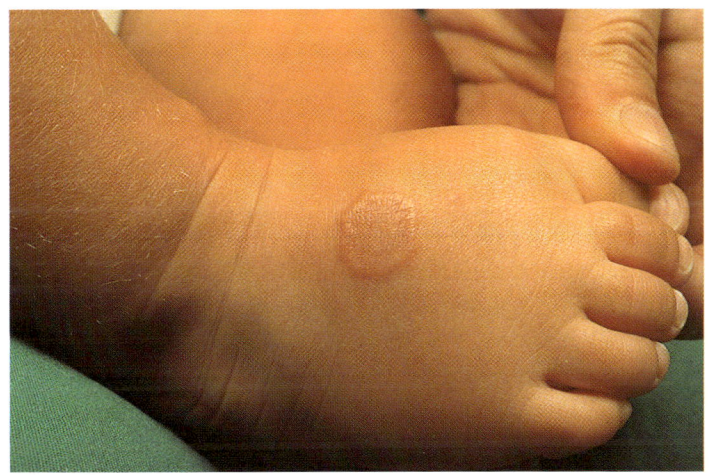

Figure 1.36
Granuloma annulare. This annular lesion comprises numerous smooth, reddish brown, firm, dome-shaped papules. The centre is depressed and macular.

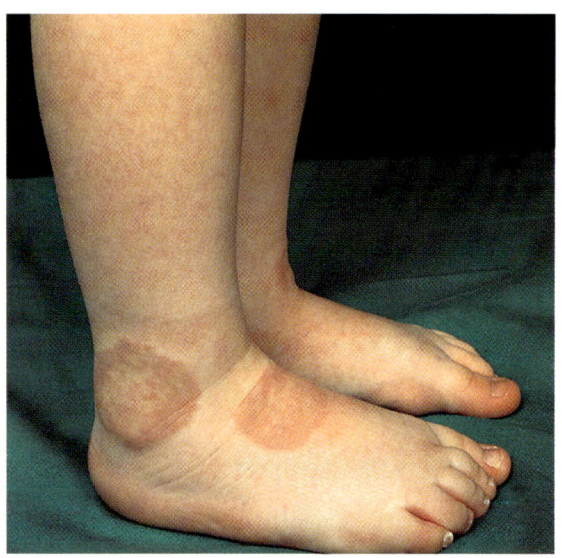

Figure 1.37
Granuloma annulare. These two sharply demarcated annular lesions have a diameter of a few centimetres. The periphery consists of reddish brown papules, the centre is depressed and skin coloured.

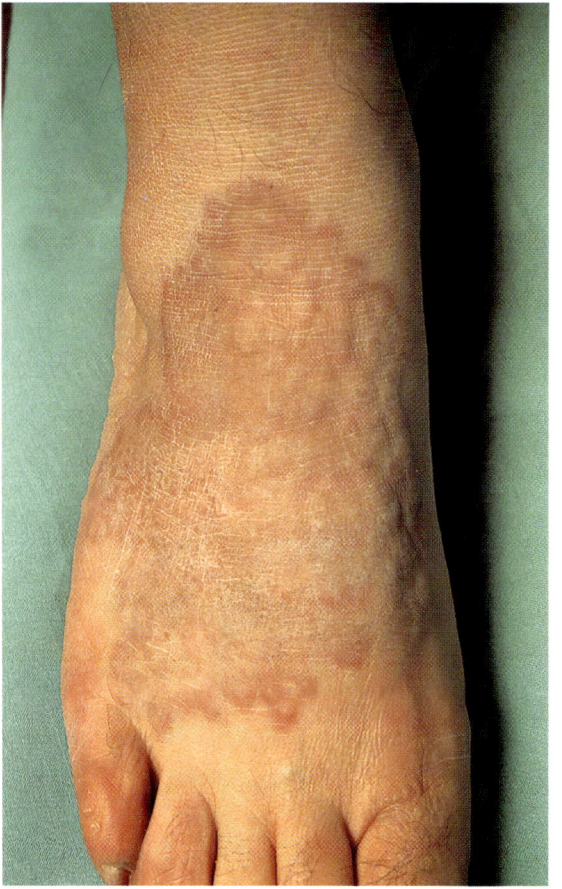

Figure 1.38
Granuloma annulare. This large lesion on the back of the foot is asymptomatic: it represents the typical, slow development of this disease.

ERYTHEMA MULTIFORME

Erythema multiforme is an acute, usually self-limit-ing, often recurrent disease that consists of the characteristic erythematous 'iris' or 'target'-shaped papules and vesicobullous lesions that are distributed symmetrically on acral sites. In severe forms the mucous membranes may be involved. Itching and burning may accompany the lesions. The disease occurs primarily in young adults between 20 and 40 years of age. An investigation for evidence of herpes virus infection or drugs is necessary.

Clinical features

The iris or target-shaped lesions are located symmetrically on the dorsal aspect of the feet or on the soles.

Differential diagnosis

Linear IgA dermatosis presents as tense bullae that have rosette or jewel-like patterns. The lesions are not symmetrically distributed.

Bullous pemphigoid is characterized by large, tense bullae that are distributed randomly and by the presence of IgG deposits along the basement membrane zone.

Dermatitis herpetiformis consists of papulovesic-ular eruptions that are always associated with a gluten-sensitive enteropathy. Granular IgA deposits are evident in the tips of the papillae. Urticaria occurs as pruritic, transient wheals.

Sweet's disease is characterized by sharply bordered inflammatory plaques and is associ-ated with fever and peripheral leucocytosis with neutrophilia.

Rowel's syndrome is a rare form of lupus erythematous; it has antinuclear antibodies and a lupus band test is positive.

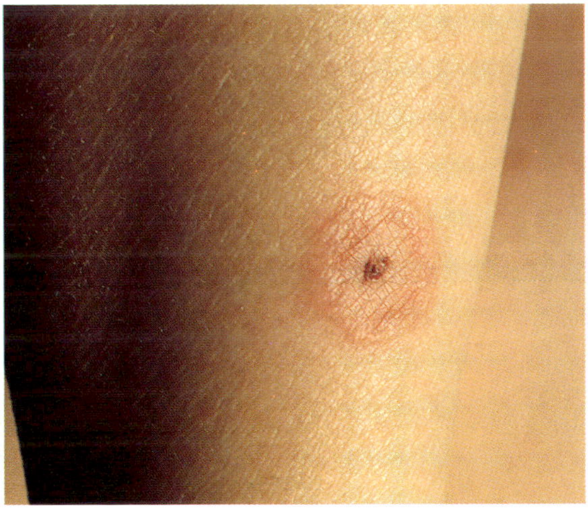

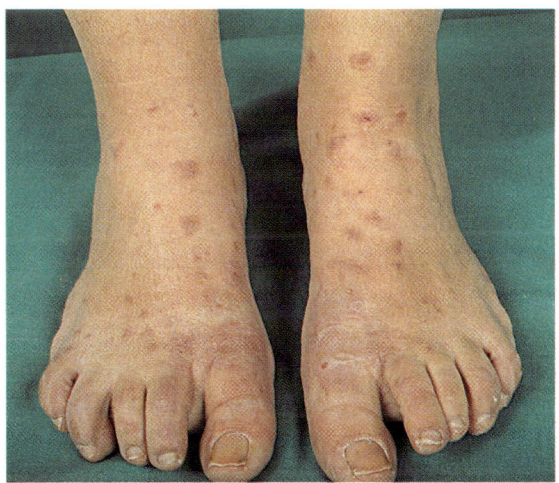

Figure 1.39
Erythema multiforme. This fully developed lesion consists of concentric rings that resemble a 'target'. At its periphery is a red vesicular rim, next to which is another pale ring; in the centre is a crust.

Figure 1.40
Erythema multiforme. In this patient the lesions appear in a symmetrical fashion.

DERMATITIS HERPETIFORMIS

Dermatitis herpetiformis (DH) is a chronic disorder associated with gluten enteropathy. It is characterized clinically by intensely pruritic papules and vesicles that tend to be grouped in a herpetiform fashion.

These lesions are distributed symmetrically over the shoulders, elbows, sacrum, buttocks and knees. The peak age of onset is the third decade of life, but the disease is sometimes observed in children. After presentation DH usually persists indefinitely. Histopathologically, it is characterized by sub-epidermal vesicles in which there are numerous neutrophils. Granular IgA deposits, detected on direct immunofluorescence in the papillary dermis of normal-appearing skin, is the most reliable method of diagnosis.

Clinical features

Infection of the feet, although rare, tends to affect the dorsal aspect.

Differential diagnosis

Nummular atopic dermatitis has a random distribution; it is not associated with gluten enteropathy and direct immunofluorescence is negative.

In contact dermatitis the lesions are not grouped in a herpetiform fashion; patch tests are positive and direct immunofluorescence is negative.

In IgA linear dermatitis the lesions are jewel-like, mainly involving the perioral and pelvic areas of the body. Gluten enteropathy is absent.

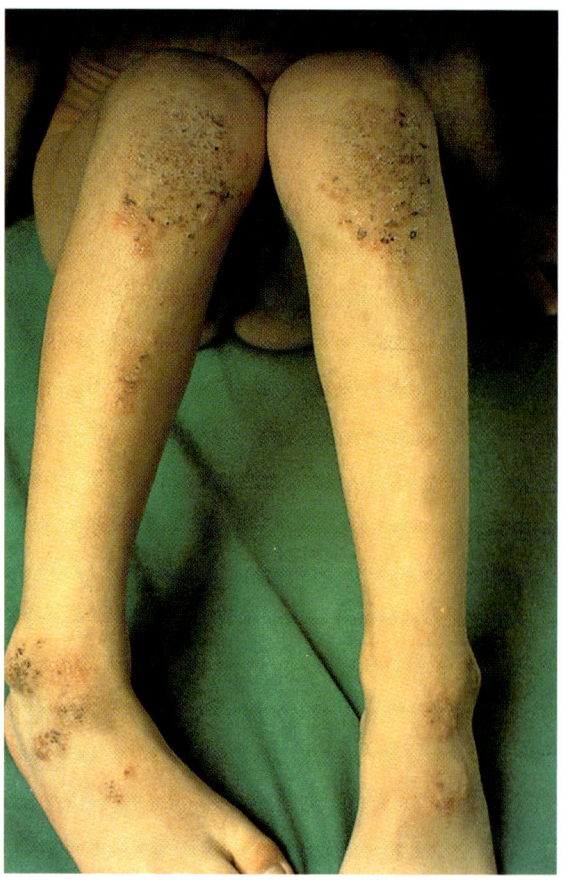

Figure 1.41
Dermatitis herpetiformis. In this young patient the lesions consist of papules and vesicles grouped in a herpetiform fashion: these are distributed symmetrically on the knees and on the dorsal aspect of the feet. Many of the lesions are eroded and crusted as a consequence of the patient having scratched them.

LINEAR IgA DERMATOSIS OF CHILDHOOD

Linear IgA dermatosis (LAD) of childhood (or chronic bullous disease of childhood) is a rare benign vesicobullous eruption. It has a typical annular pattern and mainly involves the pelvic and perioral areas of the body. Localization on the feet is unusual.

The disease's onset is during the first years of life: children are generally affected around the age of 4 years. Spontaneous regression occurs in most patients before they reach puberty. Direct immunofluorescence reveals linear IgA deposits at the dermo-epidermal junction; in approximately 60% of patients, indirect immunofluorescence demonstrates circulating IgA antibodies at the basement membrane zone.

Clinical features

There are eruptions of tense bullae that have typical rosette or jewel-like patterns. Pruritus is often present. Lesions on the feet occur as part of a more generalized eruption.

Differential diagnosis

In dermatitis herpetiformis the lesions are pruritic vesicles and a gluten-sensitive enteropathy is always present.

Impetigo may be differentiated by its yellowish crusts and by Gram stain of the contents of a pustule.

In erythema multiforme iris and target-shaped lesions are distributed symmetrically on the limbs; mucous membrane involvement is frequent.

Bullous pemphigoid requires an immunofluorescence study in order to be differentiated from LAD.

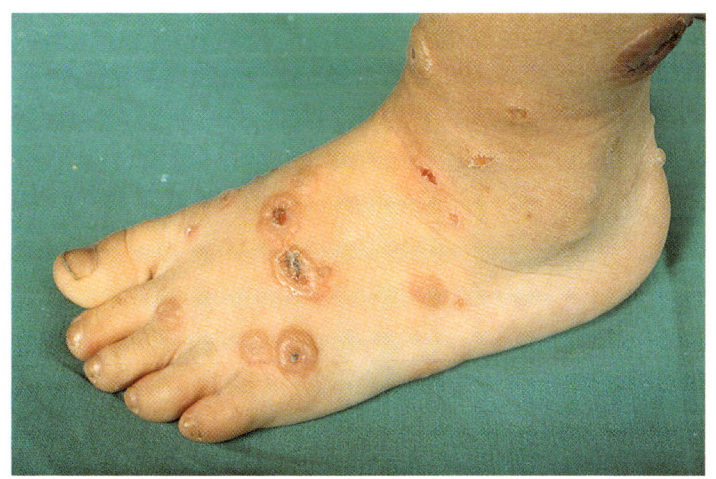

Figure 1.42(a)

Linear IgA dermatosis of childhood. On the dorsal aspect of these two children (a,b), tense vesicles are apparent in arcuate and annular configurations: these resemble rosettes.

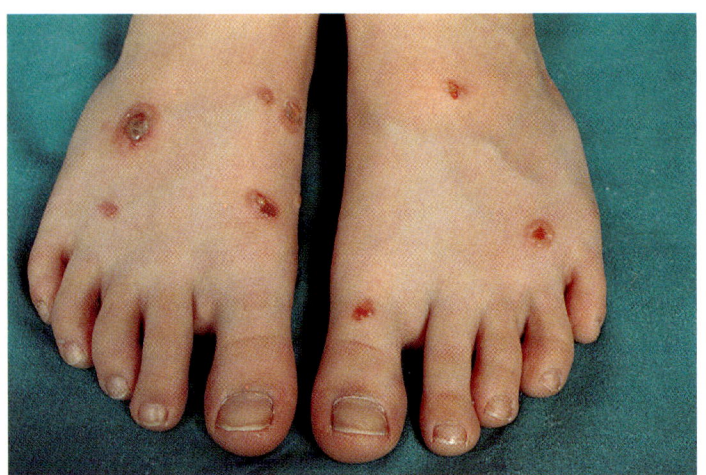

Figure 1.42(b)

Linear IgA dermatosis of childhood.

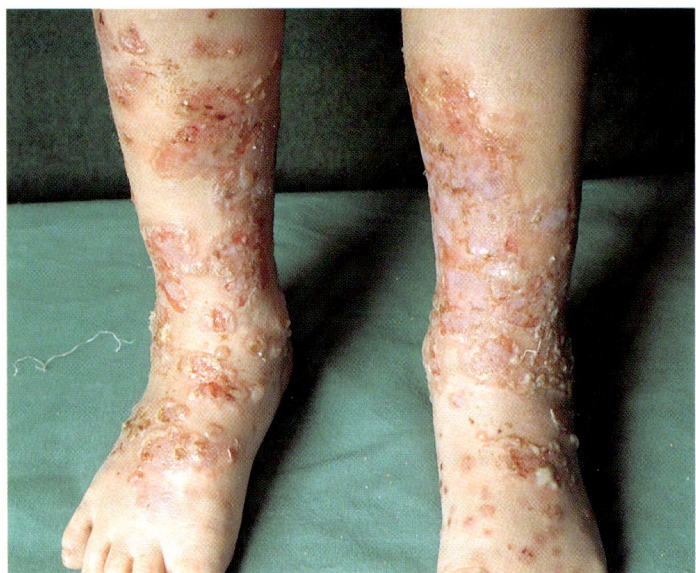

Figure 1.43

Linear IgA dermatosis of childhood. In this very aggressive example of the condition, numerous tense vesicles and bullae are present – some clustered together, others in annular array.

EPIDERMOLYSIS BULLOSA ACQUISITA

Epidermolysis bullosa acquisita (EBA) is a rare immunobullous disease characterized by:

- no family history of bullous disorders;
- a subepidermal blister demonstrated by histological examination;
- linear IgG deposits within the dermo-epidermal junction on direct immunofluorescence; and
- circulating antibodies against type VII collagen of anchoring fibrils.

EBA presents in three ways, simulating epidermolysis bullosa dystrophica, bullous pemphigoid and cicatricial pemphigoid. The age of onset is usually late in life and the course is chronic.

Clinical features

When the feet are involved this is mainly in the form simulating epidermolysis bullosa dystrophica, with blisters and erosions at the sites of trauma. The blisters may be haemorrhagic and these resolve with scarring and milia.

Differential diagnosis

The diagnostic criteria listed above allow easy differentiation from the other acquired bullous diseases, such as bullous pemphigoid and cicatricial pemphigoid. Porphyria cutanea tarda may be ruled out because of the absence of urinary porphyrins and of immune deposits.

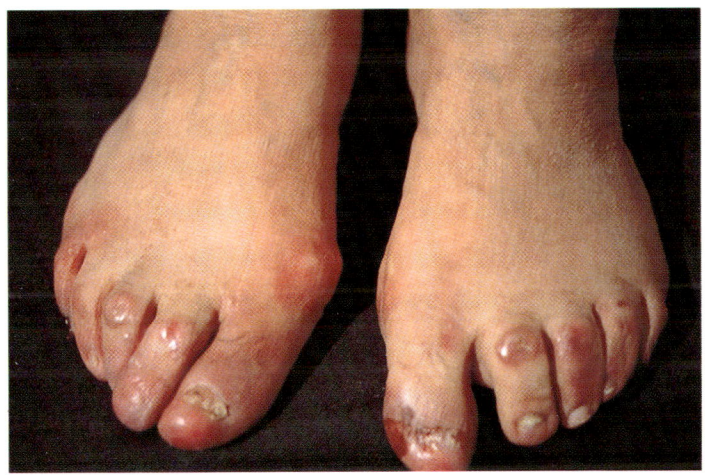

Figure 1.44

Epidermolysis bullosa acquisita. In this patient, haemorrhagic blisters, erosions covered by crusts and dystrophic nails are prominent features of the condition.

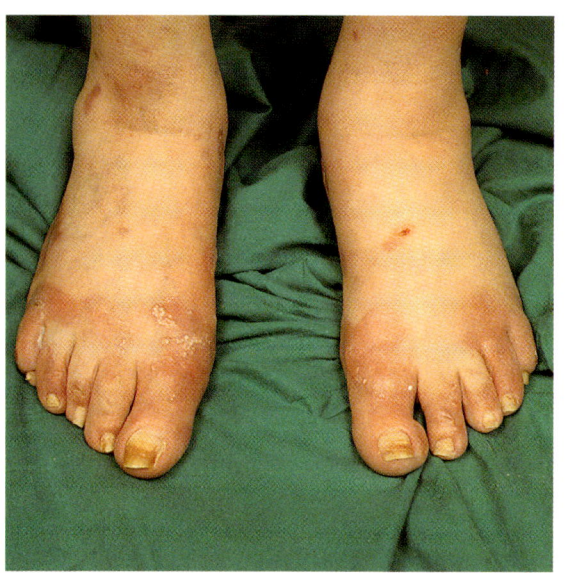

Figure 1.45

Epidermolysis bullosa acquisita. In this patient, atrophic scars and milia represent the consequence of repeated sub-epidermal blisters.

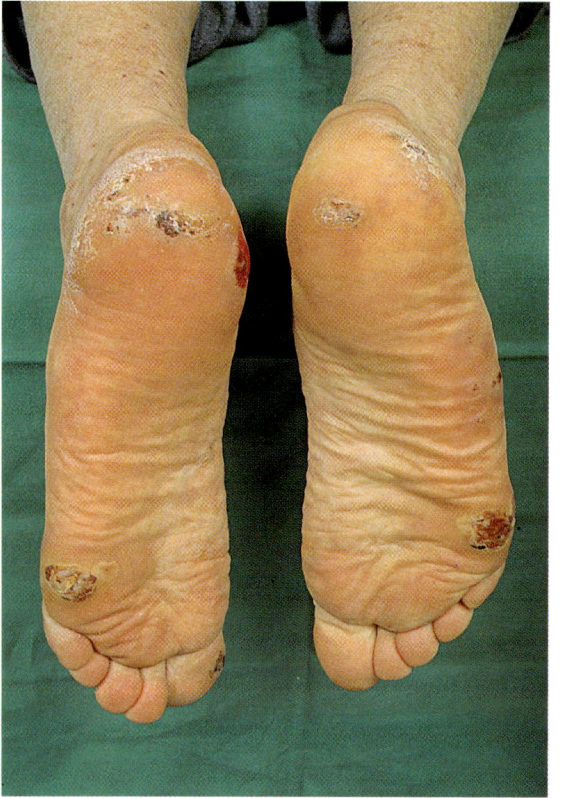

Figure 1.46

Epidermolysis bullosa acquisita. Blisters and haemorrhagic crusts are evident on the sites of major trauma.

ERYTHEMA ELEVATUM DIUTINUM

Erythema elevatum diutinum (EED) is a rare, chronic leucocytoclastic vasculitis that consists of red, purple or rust-coloured plaques located symmetrically at the elbows and knees. The lesions' distribution is highly characteristic of this disease.

The lesions have a striking predilection for the extensor surfaces of the joints of the hands, elbows and knees, but are not uncommon on the feet. The plaques are frequently depressed centrally with raised edges, and these may burn. The age of onset is usually between 30 and 60 years. The condition may be associated with dermatitis herpetiformis, inflammatory bowel diseases and myeloma or IgA gammopathies. Dapsone invokes a dramatic response in most cases.

Clinical features

The lesions are mainly located on the dorsal aspects of the feet, ankles and Achilles tendon. Nodules may be observed on the toes.

Differential diagnosis

Sweet's disease presents as tender nodules or plaques associated with fever, elevated ESR and neutrophilia, without histological evidence of severe vasculitis.

Granuloma annulare is easily differentiated by the skin-like colour of its lesions, its annular configuration – with its periphery made up of papules – and its spontaneous resolution.

Multicentric reticulohistiocytosis may be differentiated only histologically.

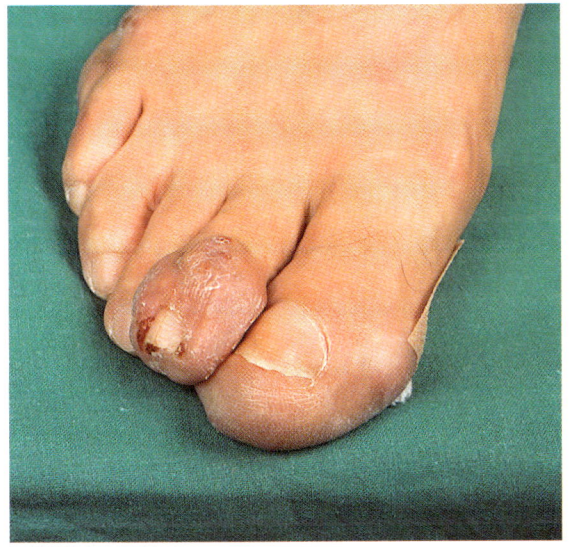
(a)

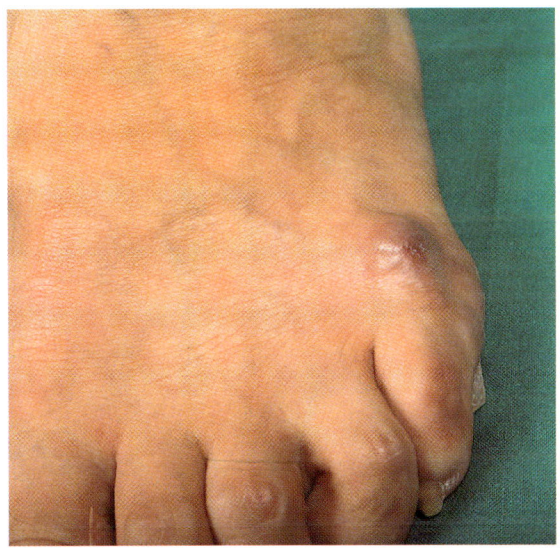
(b)

Figure 1.47(a,b)
Erythema elevatum diutinum. Reddish-purple nodules can be observed around the toes.

PYODERMA GANGRENOSUM

Pyoderma gangrenosum (PG) is an uncommon, chronic, ulcerative, non-infective skin disorder that occurs in all age groups. Its salient feature is an irregular ulcer that has a well defined, raised, undermined, erythematous to violaceous border and a 'boggy' necrotic base. These borders are often perforated and may drain pus. The lesions are usually single but may arise in clusters that coalesce. Four main variants may be distinguished: pustular, bullous, ulcerative and vegetating. The disease frequently progresses rapidly and may remain indolent for long periods; it heals leaving cribriform scars. Any area of the body may be infected but the sites of predilection are the lower legs, buttocks and abdomen. PG is confined to the skin in 50% of cases but may also be associated with inflammatory bowel diseases, leukaemia, paraproteinaemia, myeloma, arthritis and chronic hepatitis. Histopathology is not diagnostic. There is neutrophil-rich infiltration of the dermis with signs of vasculitis.

Clinical features

Eighty per cent of patients have lesions on their lower legs and the dorsal aspect of the feet. The soles are usually not involved. All variants of PD may be encountered.

Differential diagnosis

Sweet's disease is sudden in onset, is not ulcerated and is associated with fever, elevated ESR and neutrophilia.

Atypical mycobacterial infections, deep fungal infections (cryptococcosis and blastomycosis) and amoebiasis cutis may be ruled out on the basis of microbiological and histological examinations.

Allogenodermas are more hyperkeratotic.

Antiphospholipid antibody syndrome may present with pyoderma gangrenosum-like leg ulcers but may easily be differentiated through laboratory examinations.

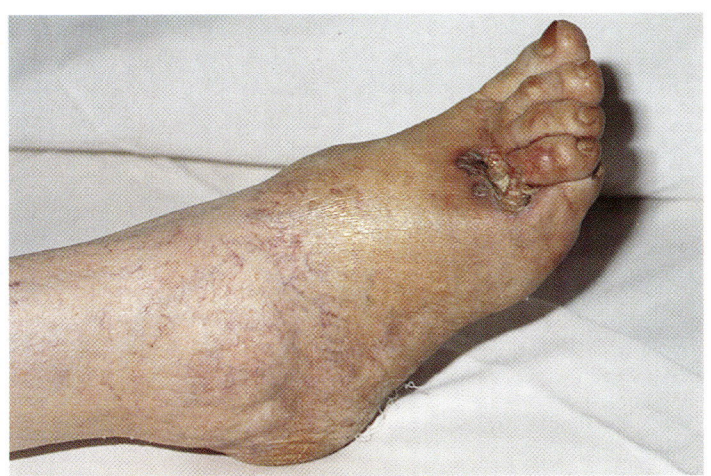

Figure 1.48

Pyoderma gangrenosum. An irregular ulcer with undermined violaceous borders and a necrotic centre is present on the distal part of the dorsal aspect of the foot.

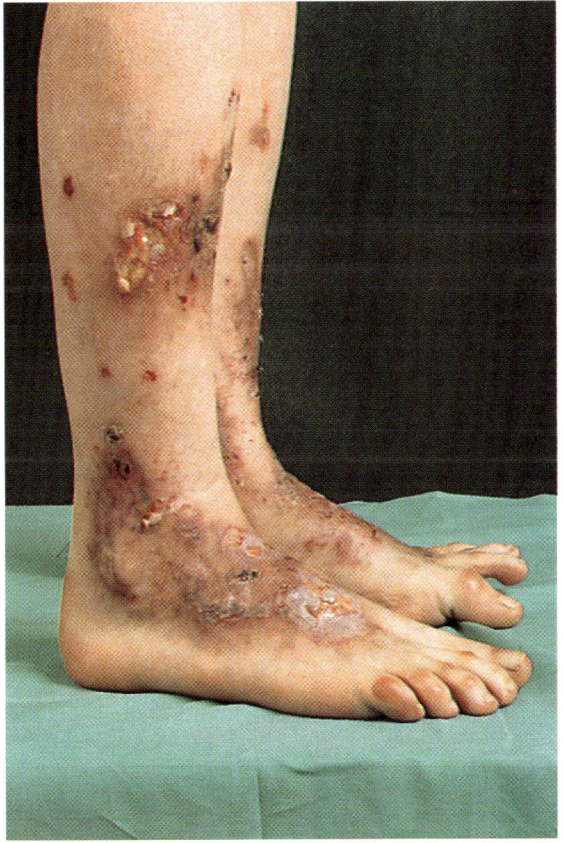

Figure 1.49

Pyoderma gangrenosum. Multiple, adjacent, indolent lesions comprising pustules, 'boggy' plaques and necrotizing ulcerations may be noted on the dorsal aspect of the foot and on the ankle.

SYSTEMIC LUPUS ERYTHEMATOSUS

Cutaneous lesions in systemic lupus erythematosus (SLE) can be classified as specific and non-specific. Specific lesions consist of the typical erythematosus malar rash which is made up of scattered maculopapular eruptions. Non-specific lesions include vasculitis, livedo reticularis, Raynaud's phenomenon and vesicobullous lesions. When these skin lesions are present, there will be strong evidence of multisystem involvement (i.e. arthritis, polyserositis and neurologic disorders). Haematological and renal involvement are common. Fever, malaise and weakness are frequent findings. Laboratory tests will provide evidence of the presence of a broad spectrum of auto-antibodies (ANA, SSA, SSB, etc.), low levels of complement and elevated ESR, haematologic abnormalities (leucopenia, anaemia, thrombocytopenia), and elevation of gammaglobulins.

Clinical features

Specific lesions on the feet are rare, and these are characterized by red to violaceous, sometimes scaling, plaques mainly localized on the toes and over the lateral borders of the feet. Of the aspecific lesions that occur on the feet, purpuric macules (as a result of thrombocytopenia of vasculitis) are the most common. Vesicles and bullae may occasionally appear on the soles and on the tips of the toes. Gangrene of the toes due to arteritis of medium-sized arteries is rare.

Differential diagnosis

Papular scaly plaques must be differentiated from lichen planus (violaceous, itching lesions) and psoriasis (scalloped margins and presence of other lesions typical of this disease).

Purpuric and necrotic lesions due to other forms of cutaneous vasculitis are ruled out by laboratory tests. Vesiculobullous lesions require differentiation from bullous lichen planus (histopathology and laboratory tests), epidermolysis bullosa acquisita (immunofluorescence) and porphyria cutanea tarda (presence of urinary prophyrins).

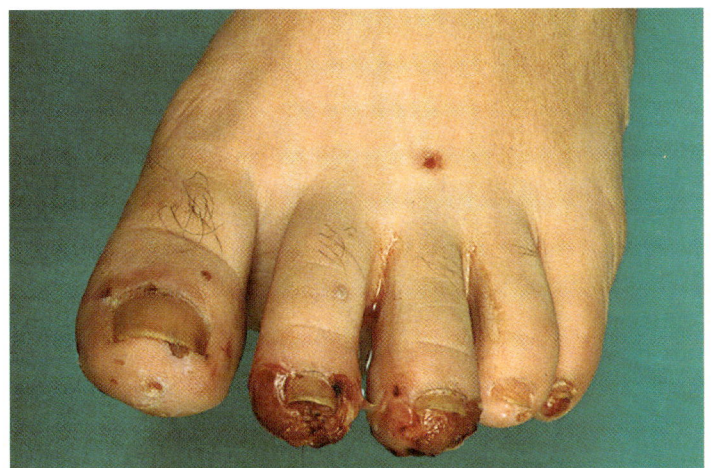

Figure 1.50

Systemic lupus erythematosus. Purpuric lesions, as a consequence of vasculitis, are a common finding on the toes in this condition.

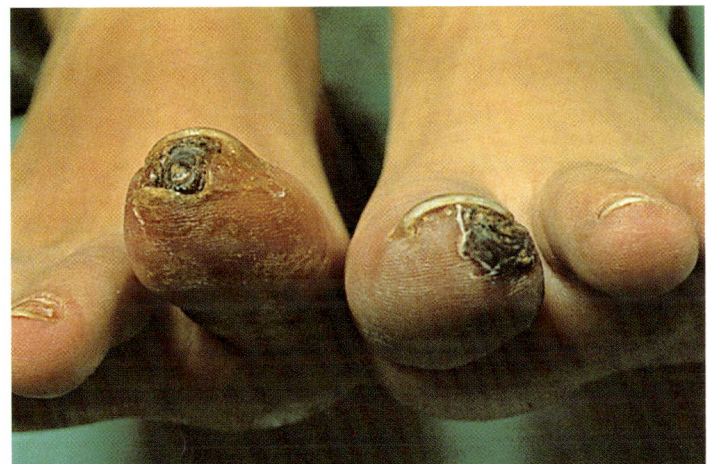

Figure 1.51

Systemic lupus erythematosus. Gangrene of the toes is a consequence of arteritis of medium-sized arteries.

CAPILLARITIS OF THE INFERIOR LIMBS

Several chronic disorders of unknown aetiology may be classified under the name of purpuric capillaritis of the inferior limbs: they are characterized clinically by purpuric lesions and histologically by endothelial swelling, extravasation of red cells and haemosiderin deposition in the macrophages.

Schamberg's dermatosis or progressive pigmented purpuric dermatosis consists of irregular reddish brown plaques that have 'cayenne pepper' spots. In pigmented purpuric lichenoid dermatosis of Gougerot and Blum, purpuric lesions are associated with lichenoid papules, while in purpura annularis telangiectodes of Majocchi the purpuric lesions assume an annular configuration.

The legs are the site most commonly affected, where the skin acquires a brown pigmentation.

Clinical features

Purpuric lesions with irregular borders or an annular configuration may occasionally be observed on the dorsal aspect of the feet and toes. The soles are spared. The purpuric lesions do not blanch when depressed with a glass slide.

Differential diagnosis

Irritant contact dermatitis is itchy, inflammatory and is rapid in onset.

Allergic contact dermatitis can be identified with patch tests.

Drug-induced vasculitides are characterized by the acute eruption of palpable purpuras. An investigation of the patient's history may identify the cause of the disease.

Dysproteinaemic and thrombocytopenic purpuras are ruled out by laboratory tests.

Henoch–Schönlein purpura is a palpable purpura that is associated with arthalgias and gastrointestinal problems.

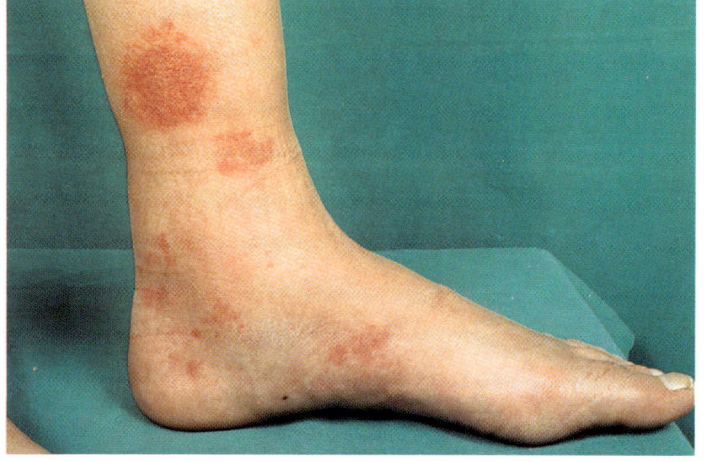

Figure 1.52
Purpuric capillaritis of the inferior limbs. Reddish-brown, irregular patches and purpuric lesions with an annular configuration are typical manifestations of this disease.

HENOCH–SCHÖNLEIN PURPURA OR ANAPHYLACTOID PURPURA

Henoch–Schönlein (H–S) is a normothrombocytic purpura that occurs mainly in children and adolescents. It is characterized clinically by a distinctive erythemato-urticarial and purpuric rash that is associated with gastrointestinal (75% of cases), joint (50%) and renal (20%) problems. The disease has an acute onset and the lesions are distributed symmetrically on the limbs, buttocks and face. The rash is usually most prominent on the lower legs. Single episodes last for a few weeks but recurrences are common in about 50% of cases. Histologically, the disease is a leukocytoclastic vasculitis with IgA deposits.

Clinical features

The dorsal aspect of the feet is the most common site, mainly affecting patients under 2 years of age. The lesions in 'palpable' purpura first appear as erythematous-oedematous macules which rapidly turn into haemorrhagic papules that are surrounded by an erythematous ring. The soles are usually spared.

Differential diagnosis

Erythema multiforme is characterized by target-like lesions that are often seen on the soles.

Gianotti–Crosti syndrome may be recognized by the typical lentil-sized papular or papulovesicular eruption that is associated with a viral infection.

Insect bites consist of asymmetrically distributed papulonodular pruritic eruptions.

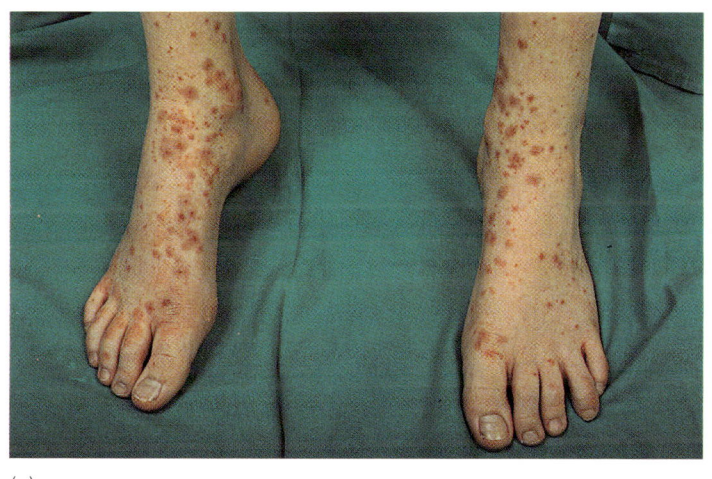

(a)

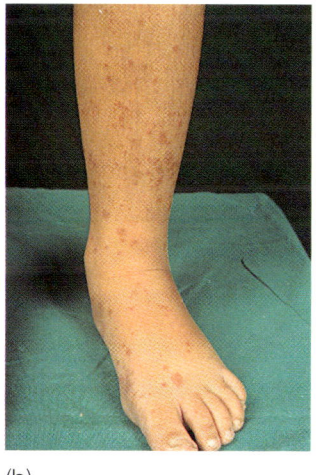

(b)

Figure 1.53(a,b)

Henoch–Schönlein purpura. Purpuric macules and papules that vary markedly in size are distributed symmetrically on the dorsal aspect of the feet of these children. Some of the lesions are haemorrhagic and are surrounded by an erythematous ring.

DYSPROTEINAEMIC PURPURA

The term 'dysproteinaemic purpuras' includes the purpuric lesions that are linked to disturbances in the plasma proteins.

Cryoglobulinaemia and hyperglobulinaemia due to underlying primary diseases, such as Waldenström's macroglobulinaemia, lupus erythematosus, sarcoidosis, rheumatoid arthritis, myeloma and Sjögren's syndrome, may induce purpura. Hyperviscosity and immuno-complex vasculitis seem to be the causative factors.

Clinical features

The lower extremities are the site of predilection. On the feet, the purpuric lesions may be observed on both the dorsum of the foot and on the soles. Necrotic lesions may occasionally appear on the toes.

Differential diagnosis

The diagnosis of dysproteinaemic purpura is based on laboratory tests.

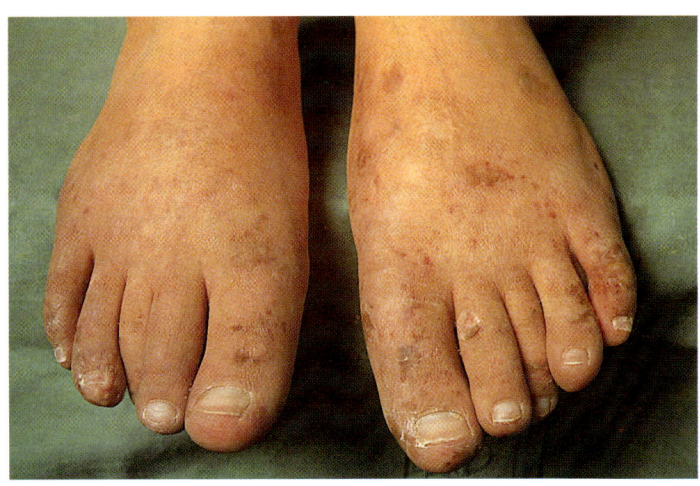

Figure 1.54(a,b)

Dysproteinaemic purpura. In this patient with Waldenström's macroglobulinaemia, purpuric lesions are present on both the dorsal aspect of the feet and on the soles.

(a)

(b)

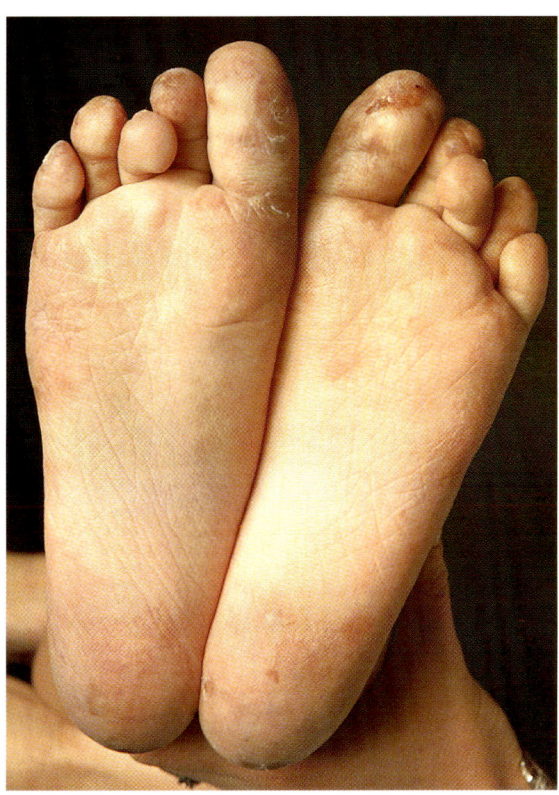

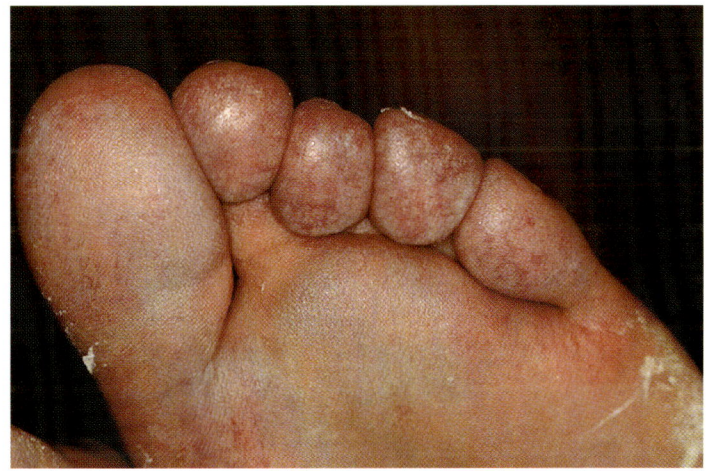

Figure 1.55

Dysproteinaemic purpura. Note the purpuric lesions on the toes of this patient with antiphospholipidic syndrome.

DRUG-INDUCED PURPURA

Drugs may cause purpuric lesions through two main mechanisms: thrombocytopenia and, most frequently, hypersensitivity vasculitis. Drug-induced purpura is a prototype of leucocytoclastic vasculitis and the main triggering factors seem to be the thiazides and carbromal. The legs and arms are most commonly infected.

Clinical features

Purpuric macules, papules and blisters are seen most frequently on the dorsal aspect of the feet where, sometimes, they tend to merge into plaques. Purpuric lesions observed on the soles are usually macular.

Differential diagnosis

Thrombocytopenic purpuras are ruled out by platelet counts.

Purpuras linked to lupus erythematosus are ruled out by laboratory tests.

Erythema multiforme is characterized by its target-like lesions.

Henoch–Schönlein purpura is most common in children and adolescents, but is not uncommon in adults; it is associated with gastrointestinal, joint and renal problems.

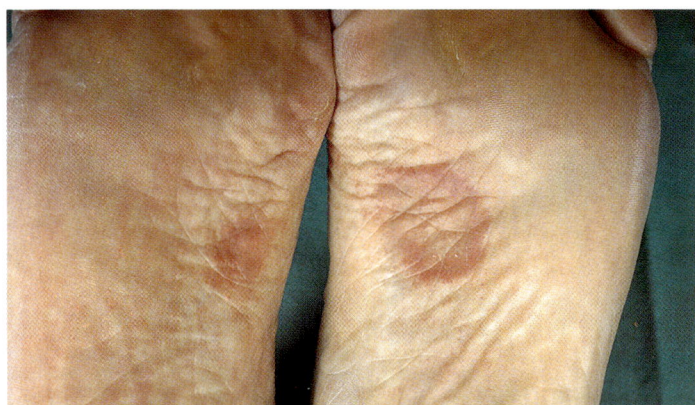

Figure 1.56
Drug-induced purpura. These plantar, purpuric patches were induced by a non-steroidal antiinflammatory drug.

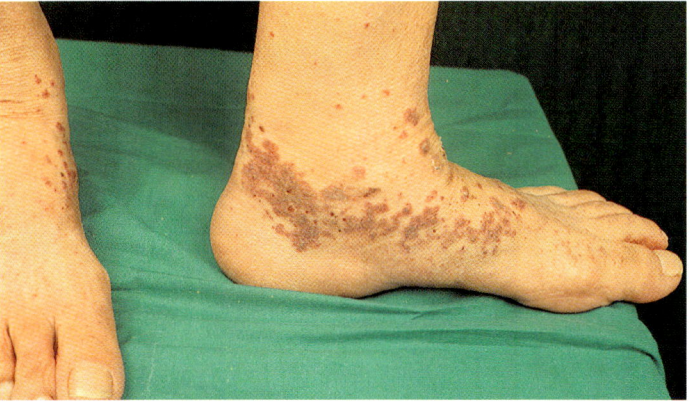

Figure 1.57
Drug-induced purpura. Purpuric papules that tend to merge into plaques are the consequence of leucocytoclastic vasculitis that was triggered by carbromal.

LOCALIZED SCLERODERMA (MORPHOEA)

Localized scleroderma is a disorder of the connective tissue that is characterized by dermal hardening on the feet. It has two main forms: plaque morphea and linear morphea.

Plaque morphea consists of round or oval, well circumscribed indurated ivory-coloured patches which, in the active phase, are surrounded by a violaceous rim (lilac ring). There is associated alopecia within the lesions.

Linear morphea appears first as an erythematous, usually asymmetric patch that, within weeks, evolves into a waxy sclerotic, band-like lesion. The lilac ring is generally absent. These lesions tend to involve the underlying tissues (scleroatrophy), producing severe malformations. Both plaque and linear morphea are seen on the dorsal aspect of the feet.

Differential diagnosis

Plaque morphea is readily distinguished from lichen sclerosus et atrophicus because of the absence of hyperkeratosis and follicular plugs.

Skin atrophy following intradermal injections of steroids will have a history of previous injections and is characterized by atrophy, not by hardening.

Linear morphea may resemble a partial lipoatrophy, but in this case there is a loss of subcutaneous tissue over a normal epidermis.

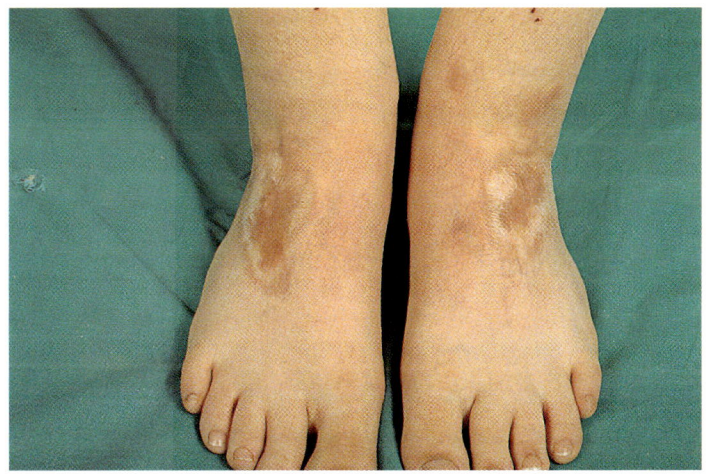

Figure 1.58
Plaque morphea. On the dorsal aspect of the feet are two symmetrical, irregularly shaped plaques that consist of a central zone of hyperpigmentation surrounded by a whitish, sclerotic halo.

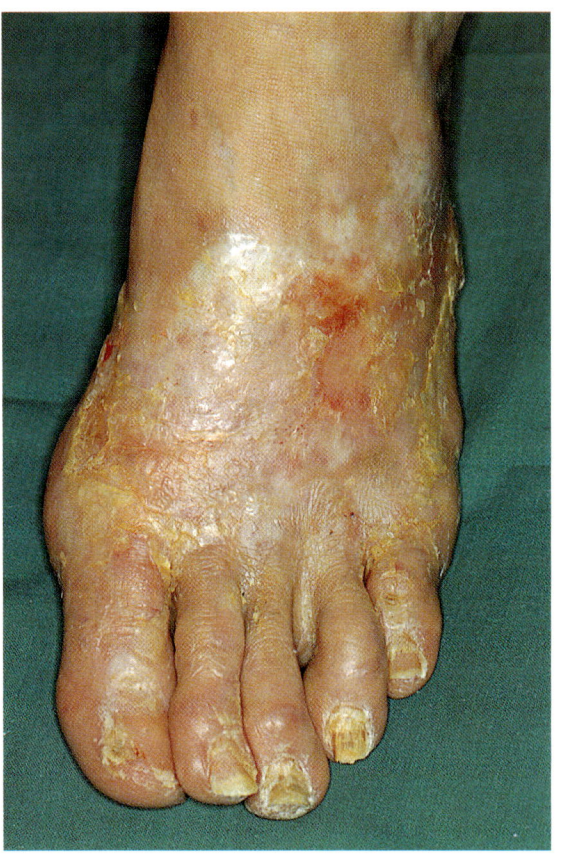

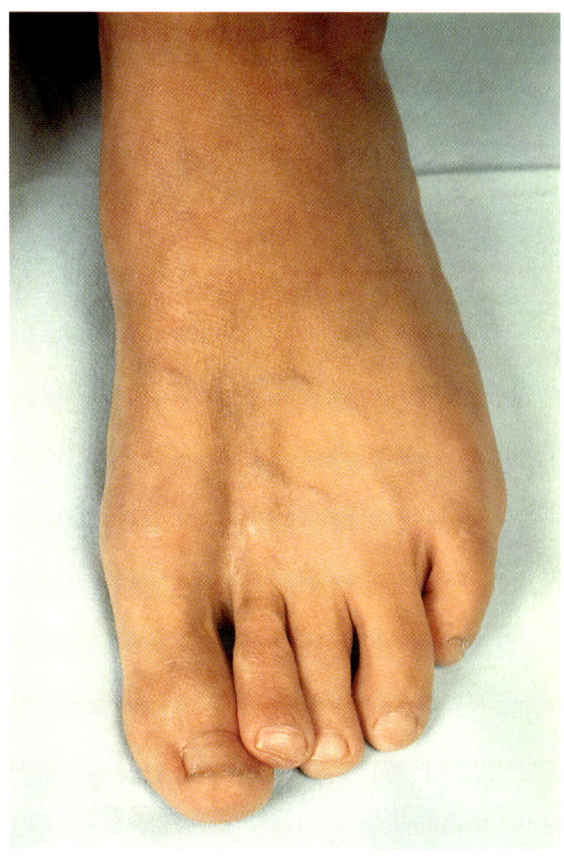

Figure 1.59

Plaque morphea. This old sclerotic lesion on the back of the foot is characterized by an alopecic, ivory-coloured patch that has ill-defined scaly borders. (Photograph courtesy of Professor Aldo Finzi.)

Figure 1.60

Linear morphea. This depressed-band lesion is a result of involvement of the underlying tissue.

LICHEN SCLEROSUS ET ATROPHICUS

Lichen sclerosus et atrophicus (LSA) is an uncommon chronic mucocutaneous disorder that is characterized by atrophy in the genital area and white papular lesions on the rest of the skin.

Extragenital lesions are distinctive, asymptomatic, ivory-white, shiny, well defined, round or polygonal firm papules a few millimetres in diameter. Their surface typically displays dilated orifices often containing horny plugs (follicular hyperkeratosis). If plugging is marked, the surface appears verrucous. These papules usually aggregate into plaques, with 'cigarette paper' atrophy. The sites of predilection are the upper part of the trunk, the neck and the upper extremities. The disease frequently appears before 7 years of age. The most striking histological finding is a band of hyalinization of the dermal collagen below the epidermis.

Clinical features

Occasionally, typical porcelain-white papular lesions may be observed on the ankles and on the dorsal aspect of the feet. The sole is only very rarely affected. The papules are hyperkeratotic and are easier to see on the weight-bearing surface of the foot. The form of LSA that exclusively involves the palms and soles is extremely rare.

Differential diagnosis

Lichen planus is easily distinguished by its itchy, violaceous papules. The characteristic papules with their follicular plugs permit differentiation from morphea.

Plantar lesions need to be differentiated from punctata keratoderma and the pits of Darier's disease. In these cases histopathology is necessary.

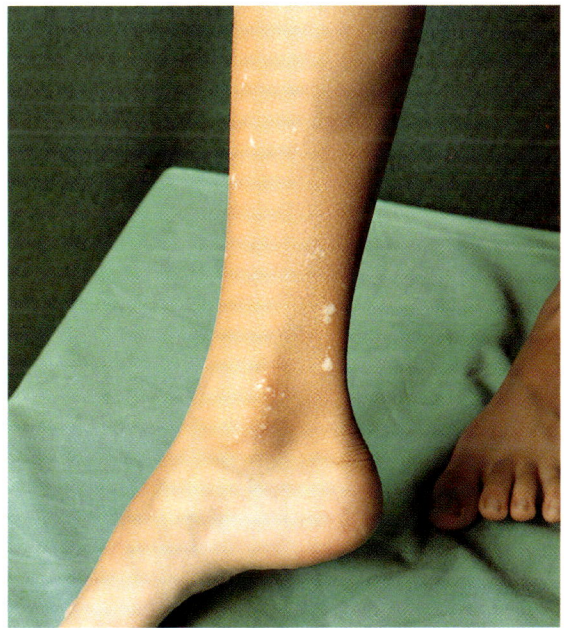

Figure 1.61
Lichen sclerosus et atrophicus. Ivory-white, shiny, well defined, round, firm papules are present on the ankle of this patient.

2 Proliferative diseases

INFANTILE DIGITAL FIBROMATOSIS
ACQUIRED DIGITAL FIBROKERATOMA
KNUCKLE PADS
KOENEN'S TUMOUR
PLANTAR FIBROMATOSIS
HYPERTROPHIC SCARS AND KELOIDS
PROTEUS SYNDROME
JUVENILE HYALINE FIBROMATOSIS
DERMOCHONDROCORNEAL DYSTROPHY
FIBROHISTIOCYTOMA AND DERMATOFIBROMA
HEMANGIOMAS
PORT-WINE STAIN
MIBELLI'S ANGIOKERATOMA
ANGIOKERATOMA CIRCUMSCRIPTUM
PYOGENIC GRANULOMA
BLUE RUBBER-BLEB NAEVI SYNDROME
KAPOSI'S SARCOMA
BLUEFARB–STEWART SYNDROME
LYMPHANGIOMA CIRCUMSCRIPTUM
ECCRINE POROMA
BOWEN'S DISEASE
KERATOACANTHOMA
SQUAMOUS CELL CARCINOMA
NAEVOID BASAL-CELL CARCINOMA SYNDROME
CONGENITAL MELANOCYTIC NAEVI
ACQUIRED MELANOCYTIC NAEVI
PEUTZ–JEGHERS SYNDROME
MALIGNANT MELANOMA
LANGERHANS' CELL HISTIOCYTOSIS
JUVENILE XANTHOGRANULOMA
MASTOCYTOSIS
SARCOMAS
MYCOSIS FUNGOIDES
METASTASIS OF THE TOES

INFANTILE DIGITAL FIBROMATOSIS

Infantile digital fibromatosis (IDF) (or recurring digital fibroma) is a fibrous growth characterized by single or multiple nodules on the fingers or toes of infants and children. The disease may be present at birth or can appear within the first year of life. Spontaneous remission is common. Histologically, lesions are constituted of interwoven fascicles of fibrous tissue that are characterized by numerous plump, oval fibrocytes and coarse, wiry bundles of collagen which are distributed throughout the dermis and the subcutaneous fat.

Clinical features

IDF manifests as firm, dome-shaped or bulbous nodules that are mainly located on the distal phalanges of the toes. These range in colour from that of skin through pink to red. Typically, the great toe is spared. These lesions usually cause no discomfort.

Differential diagnosis

Dermatofibroma is rare in children and is uncommon on the toes.

Koenen's tumour (periungual fibroma) is an excrescence that resembles a clove of garlic. It arises beside or beneath a nail rather than at the sides of the toes.

Supernumerary digit is very hard and often bilateral.

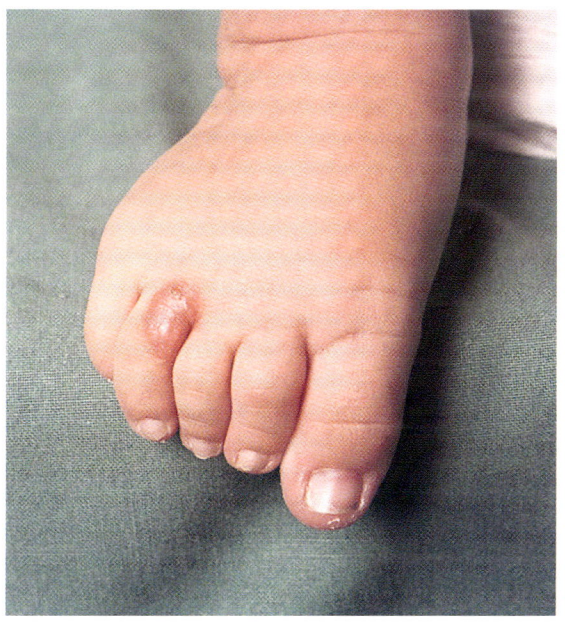

Figure 2.1

Infantile digital fibromatosis. This reddish-brown, firm, dome-shaped nodule was present at birth. The lesion disappeared spontaneously at the age of 4 years.

ACQUIRED DIGITAL FIBROKERATOMA

Acquired digital fibrokeratoma is a benign acquired fibroepithelial tumour usually located on the fingers and toes. It occurs in adults and may be preceded by trauma. Histologically it is characterized by a proliferation of connective tissue under papillomatous acanthotic and orthokeratic epidermis.

Clinical features

This is a solitary, asymptomatic, flesh-coloured, firm, dome-shaped tumour, 3–15 mm in diameter with slightly raised skin at its base. It is localized on the toes and occasionally on the soles. The lesion may be slightly warty and pedunculated.

Differential diagnosis

Infantile digital fibromatosis can be present at birth or can appear before the age of 2 years.

Koenen's tumour occurs at puberty in patients with tuberous sclerosis, emerging from the nail-bed and folds.

Supernumerary digit is usually bilateral.

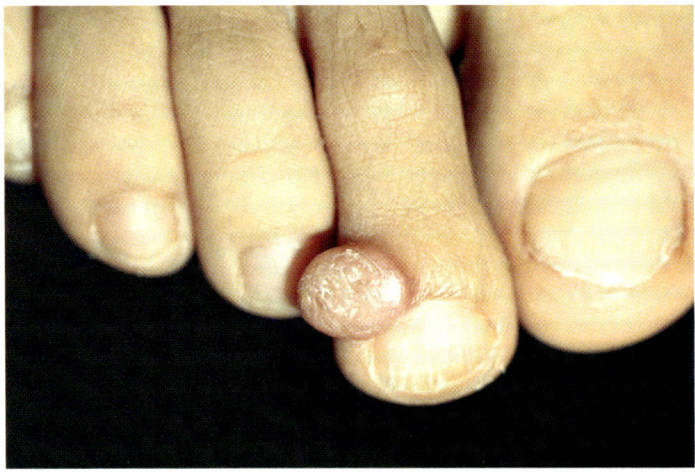

Figure 2.2
Acquired digital fibrokeratoma.
This solitary, asymptomatic, firm, flesh-coloured, dome-shaped tumour was a consequence of trauma. The top of the lesion is hyperkeratotic.

KNUCKLE PADS

Knuckle pads are well demarcated, skin-coloured, asymptomatic, smooth, hyperkeratotic nodules overlying the finger joints. These lesions rarely occur on the toes. Knuckle pads appear most frequently after the fourth decade of life. These lesions are not related to trauma and may be familial.

Differential diagnosis

Callosities are induced by trauma.
  Xanthomas are softer and yellowish.
  Warts are hyperkeratotic, irregular lesions.
  Digital mixoid cysts are solitary, firm, translucent lesions that occur at the distal interphalangeal joint of a toe.

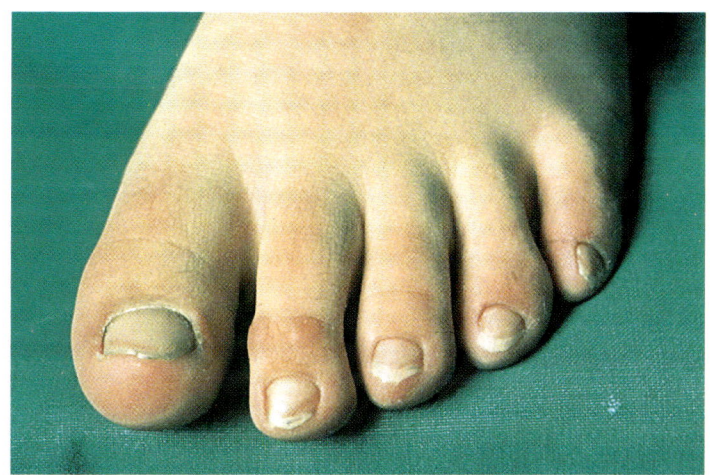

Figure 2.3

Knuckle pads. Skin-coloured, asymptomatic, smooth, slightly hyperkeratotic nodules overlie the last joint of the second toe. In this case the lesion was familial.

KOENEN'S TUMOUR

Koenen's tumours are typical periungual fibromas that occur at puberty in 50% of patients who have tuberous sclerosis. They manifest as flesh-coloured, elongated excrescences that emerge from the nail-bed and folds. Other skin lesions characteristic of tuberous sclerosis are facial angiofibromas, shagreen patches and ash-leaf white macules.

Histologically, they present as polypoid lesions covered with a normal cornified layer, and are composed of thick, bundles of collagen accompanied by an increased number of fibrocytes.

Differential diagnosis

Infantile digital fibromatosis can be present at birth or may appear before the age of 2 years. It is characterized by dome-shaped nodules located on the dorsolateral aspects of digits.

Supernumerary digit is very hard and often bilateral.

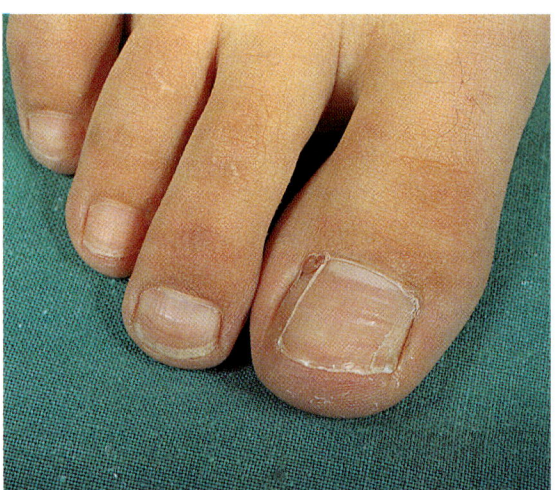

(a)

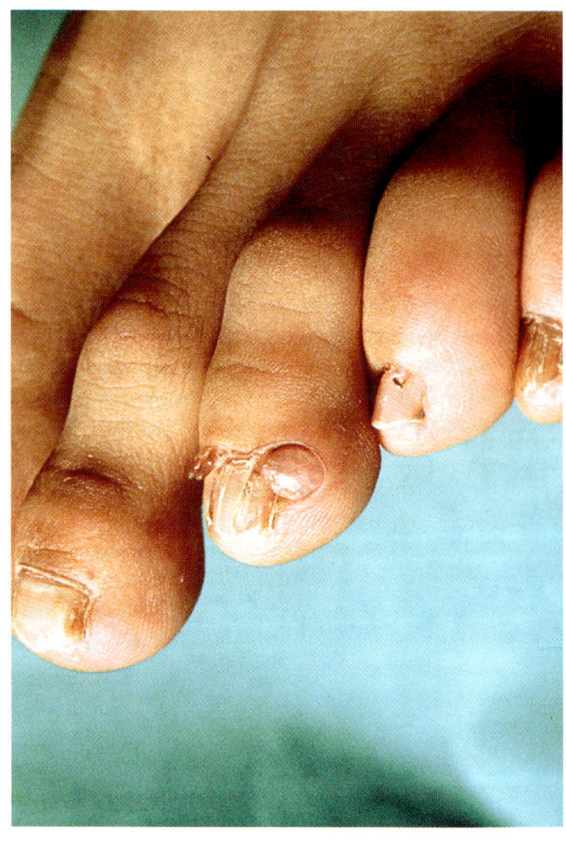

(b)

Figure 2.4(a,b)
Koenen's tumour. Somewhat warty, firm papules may be present beneath the nail-plates (a) or at their sides (b). As a consequence of their shape, these tumours have also been called 'clove of garlic tumours'.

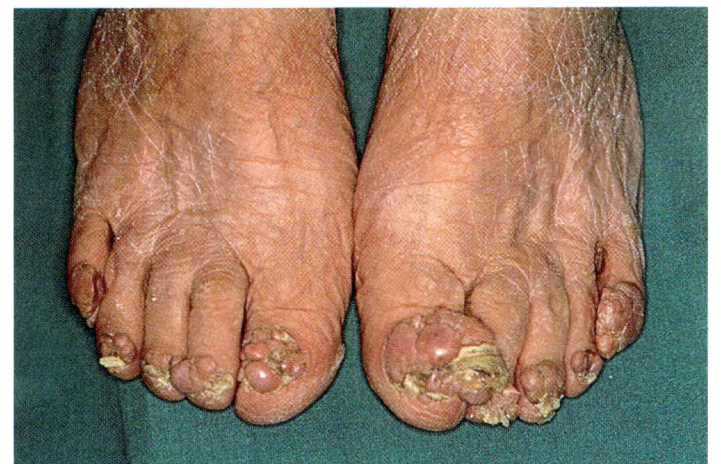

Figure 2.5(a,b)

Koenen's tumour. Reddish-brown, dome-shaped or multilobulated tumours very occasionally invade all the toes (a) and destroy nail-plates (b). (Photograph courtesy of Professor Nicola Aste.)

(a)

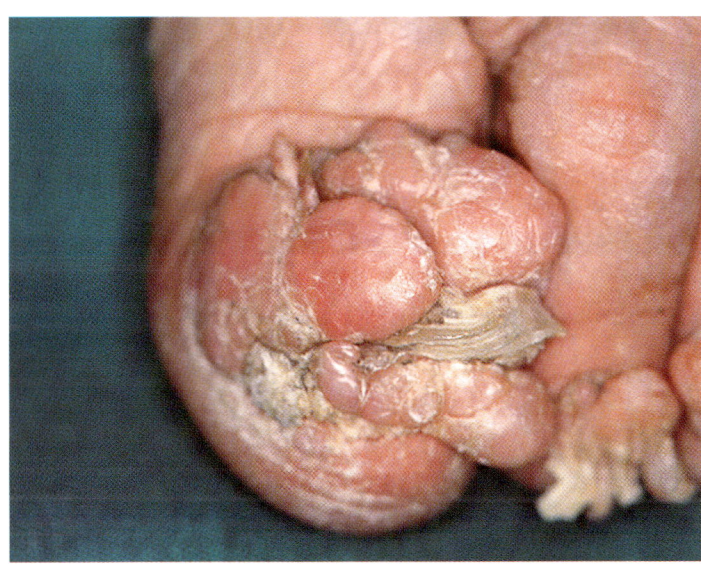

(b)

PLANTAR FIBROMATOSIS

Plantar fibromatosis is a rare condition characterized by one or more insidious, asymptomatic, firm, flesh-coloured, smooth, well-demarcated nodules that vary in diameter from a few millimetres to 4 cm. These lesions tend to be locally invasive and recur easily.

Differential diagnosis

On the soles, keloids are usually a consequence of trauma and are pink or red in colour.

Fibrosarcoma is a reddish or purplish nodule that soon ulcerates; histopathology is necessary.

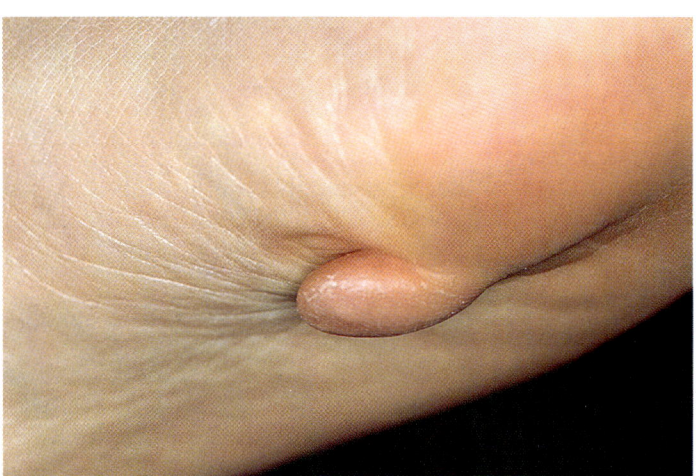

Figure 2.6

Plantar fibromatosis. This pedunculated, flesh-coloured, smooth, asymptomatic nodule was present at birth. The lesion recurred after surgical excision.

HYPERTROPHIC SCARS AND KELOIDS

Hypertrophic scars are fibrosing inflammations that remain localized to the site of injury. Keloids, which are also a fibrosing inflammation, on the other hand, extend beyond the site of injury. Both these lesions, which usually appear within a few months following a penetrating injury, are elevated and smooth surfaced. Hypertrophic scars are well defined, whereas keloids are often not. The size and appearance of the lesions may or may not be related to the underlying trauma. New lesions may be mildly erythematous in colour, whereas older lesions are pale, or occasionally hyperpigmented.

Keloids may occur anywhere but are exceedingly uncommon on the soles. However, when they do occur they may cause serious functional disability. A familial predilection to keloids is a well-established observation.

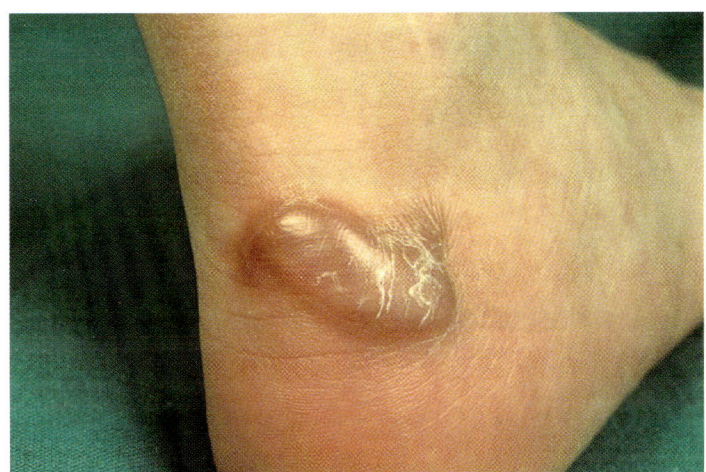

Figure 2.7

Keloids. This irregular, firm, reddish-brown, elevated, slightly scaling, fibrosing tumour appeared after trauma to the posterior side of the heel.

PROTEUS SYNDROME

Proteus syndrome is a rare hamarthomatous disorder characterized by multifocal overgrowths that can involve any part of the body. The clinical features of this disease include progressive and asymmetrical megalodactyly, hemihypertrophy, subcutaneous masses, localized cerebroid thickening of the palms and soles, and linear skin lesions. The subcutaneous masses may consist of various combinations of adipose, lymphatic and haemangiomatous tissue.

Clinical features

Cerebriform or nodular, gross thickening of the soles (and palms) is the most typical, frequent feature of this disorder.

Megalodactyly is progressive and asymmetric; syndactyly may also be observed.

Linear epidermal naevi may be present.

Differential diagnosis

Neurofibromatosis may grow asymmetrically and cause macrodactyly, but its axillary freckling and iris nodules are distinctive features of this condition.

Klippel–Trenaunay–Weber syndrome and congenital lymphoedema may lead to hypertrophy and macrodactyly, but lack the cerebriform thickening of the soles.

Maffucci's syndrome may be distinguished by the presence of enchondromatosis.

The plantar superficial fibromatosis of Ledderhose mainly occurs in males. It is characterized by asymptomatic, well defined, firm but not inflammatory nodules that are distributed bilaterally on the soles.

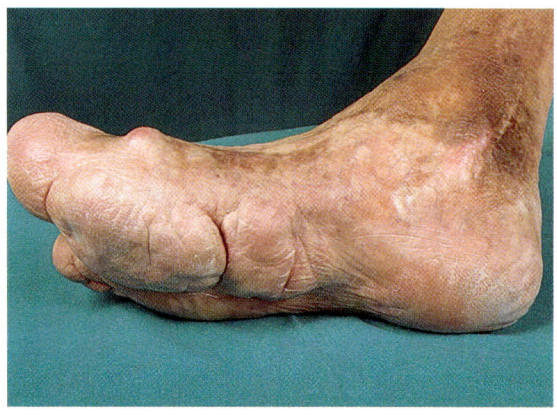

(a)

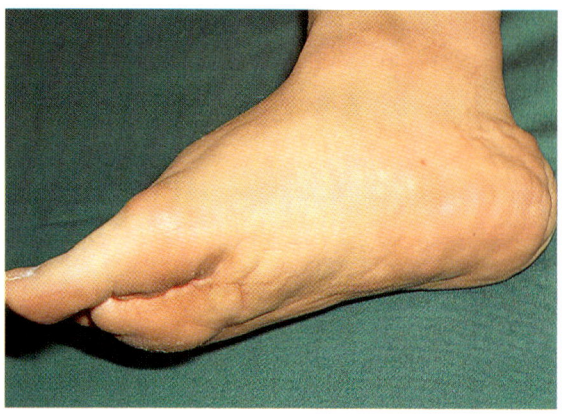

(b)

Figure 2.8(a,b)

Proteus syndrome. Cerebriform thickening of the soles, as a result of various combinations of adipose, lymphatic and angiomatous tissue, is the most frequent observation in this disease.

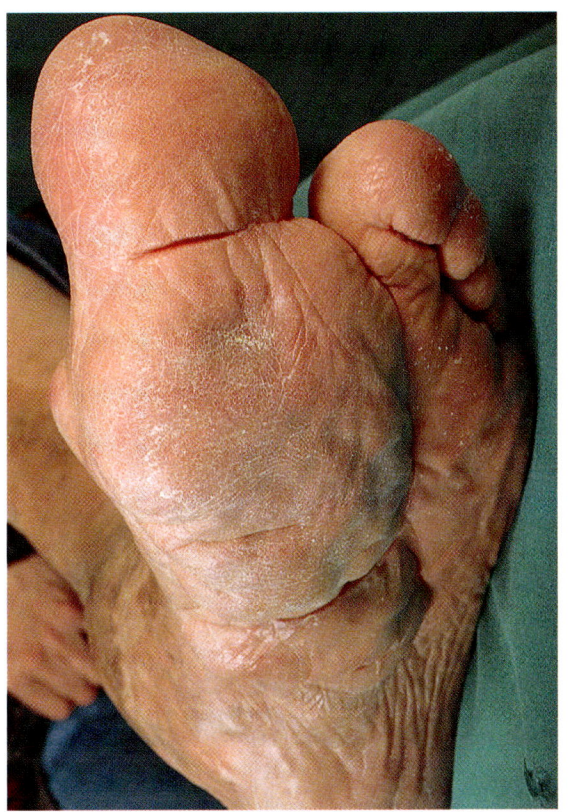

Figure 2.9

Proteus syndrome. Macrodactylia is an important finding in this disease. It is progressive and asymmetrical.

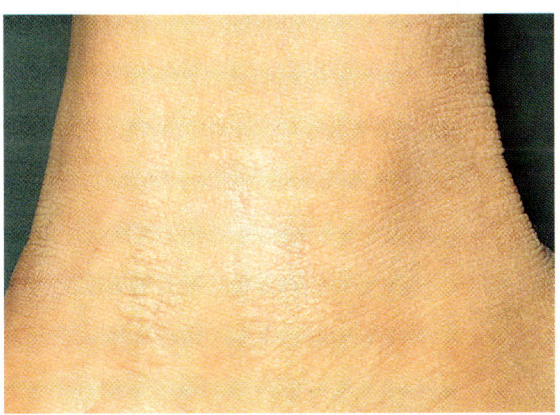

Figure 2.10

Proteus syndrome. Linear, hypopigmented, verrucous bands distributed along Blaschko's lines can be observed on the lower limb.

JUVENILE HYALINE FIBROMATOSIS

Juvenile hyaline fibromatosis (JHF) is a very rare disease characterized by numerous papules and nodules that have unique histologic features: hypertrophic gingivae, osteolytic bone lesions and deforming contractures. Three main types of skin lesions may be present:

- small, fleshy, pearly papules (mainly located on the face and neck);
- pink to violet, translucent nodules (mainly affecting the fingers and feet);
- subcutaneous nodules of variable appearance on the trunk and extremities.

The disease occurs sporadically and during the first months of life. Its course is dramatically progressive, disabling and disfiguring, but mental development is normal. Histologically the lesions are characterized by closely packed thick bundles of collagen, abundant homogenous eosinophilic material (PAS positive and diastase-resistant), and an increased presence of spindle-shaped fibroblasts that have a chondroid appearance.

Clinical features

On plantar regions, the lesions are predominantly translucent nodules. These tumours and osteolytic lesions of the phalanges cause progressive malformations.

Differential diagnosis

The triad of cutaneous lesions, gingival hypertrophy and flexural contractures allows easy differentiation from infantile myofibromatosis, generalized scleroderma, dermochondrodysplasia (Francois' syndrome) and multicentric reticulohistiocytosis.

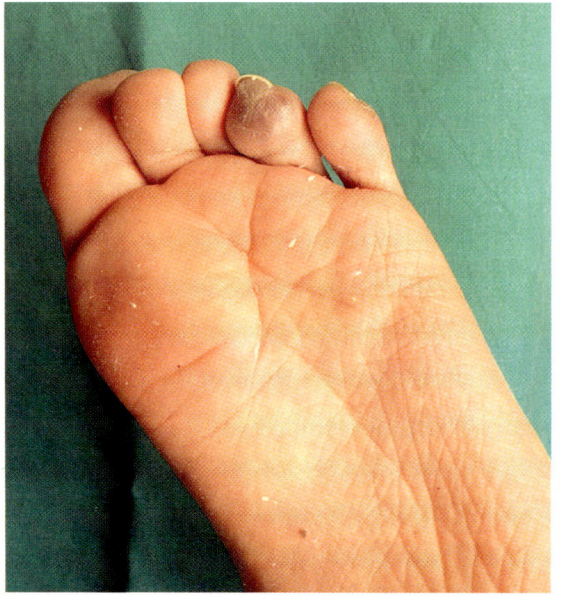

Figure 2.11
Juvenile hyaline fibromatosis. A violaceous nodule has invaded the plantar surface of a toe.

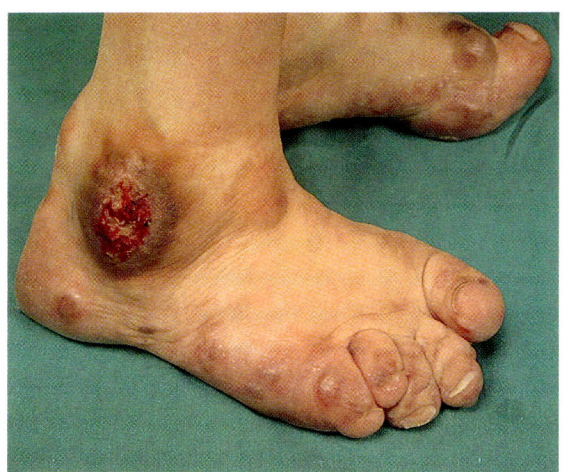

(a)

Figure 2.12(a–c)

Juvenile hyaline fibromatosis. The feet of this patient demonstrate this condition dramatically. Subcutaneous nodules are evident on the ankles, dorsal surfaces and soles of the feet. Pink, translucent nodules mainly affect the toes.

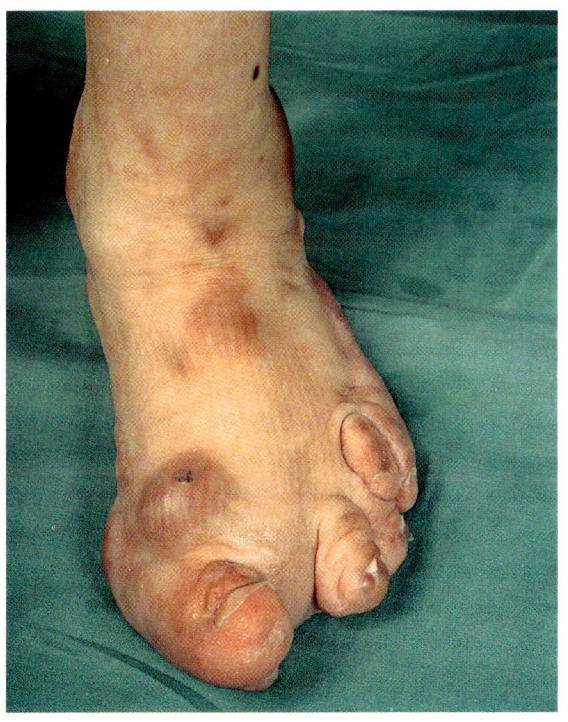

(b)

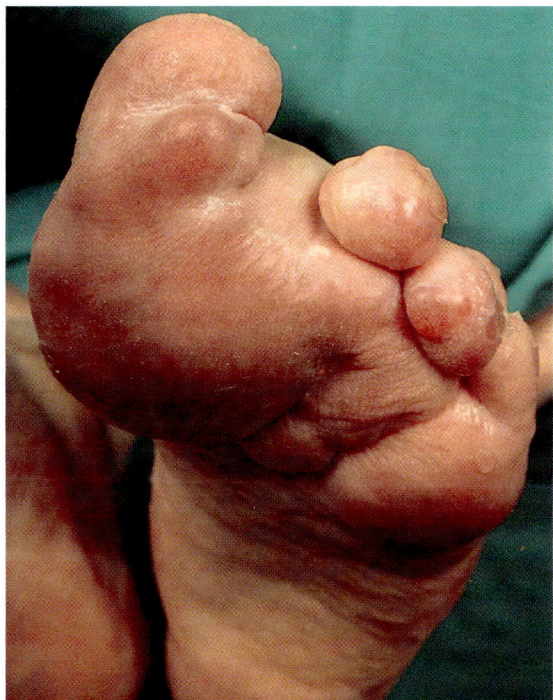

(c)

DERMOCHONDRO-CORNEAL DYSTROPHY

Dermochondrocorneal dystrophy or Francois' syndrome is an extremely rare disease characterized by firm, nodular lesions that involve the face, hands and feet. There is osteochondrodystrophy of the peripheral, extremital bones, resulting in limited movement and corneal dystrophy. Involvement of the gingival and palatal mucous membranes has been reported occasionally. The disease usually appears during childhood. Histologically, the skin lesions demonstrate abundant, vacuolated cells (spongiocytes) in the papillary and mid-dermis. There is new collagen formation, which is arranged into large, variously orientated bundles.

Clinical features

Papulonodular, white to grey or xanthoma-like lesions are mainly located on the toes. The nails may be convex.

Differential diagnosis

Familial histiocytic dermoarthritis is transmitted as an autosomal dominant trait and is characterized by both skin and joint lesions but not corneal lesions.

Fibroblastic rheumatism is a non-familial disease characterized by polyarthritis, sclerodactyly and multiple nodules distributed on the extremities. Corneal dystrophy is absent.

Juvenile hyaline fibromatosis is characterized by numerous dermal or subcutaneous nodules, flexion contractures, osteolytic bone lesions and hypertrophic gingivae.

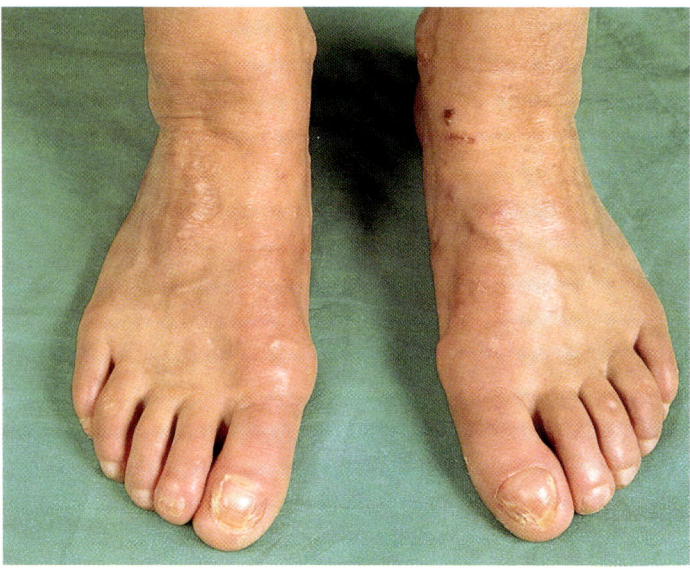

Figure 2.13
Dermochondrocorneal dystrophy. Small, whitish-grey nodules have invaded the toes. Many of the nail-plates are convex in shape.

FIBROHISTIOCYTOMA AND DERMATOFIBROMA

Fibrohistiocytoma and dermatofibroma are indicative of the same lesion at different states of evolution (highly cellular or less cellular and more fibrous). The lesions consist of well demarcated, usually asymptomatic papules or nodules that range in size from a few millimetres to 2 cm. Their colour ranges from pink to red (highly cellular lesion) to dark brown (less cellular and more fibrous). They are hard and feel like a pea or a small button attached to the skin's surface.

These tumours are mainly located on the extremities but rarely may also be seen on the soles. They generally appear within weeks or months following trauma.

Differential diagnosis

When pink or red, fibrohistiocytoma may be misinterpreted as an haemangioma or a Spitz naevi; when purple as a nodule of Kaposi's sarcoma; and when brown as a melanocytic naevus or a malignant melanoma. Histopathologic examination is frequently necessary for correct diagnosis.

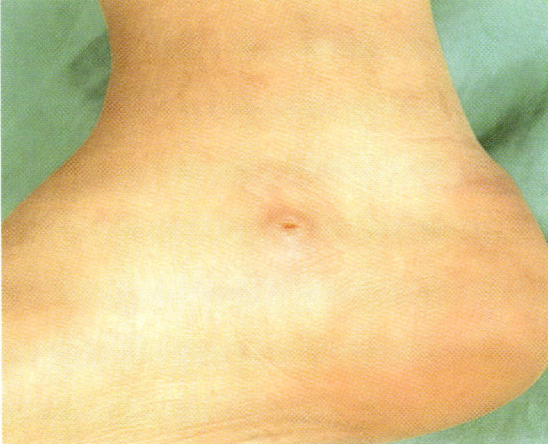

Figure 2.15
Fibrohistiocytoma and dermatofibroma. The brownish colour of this well-demarcated, firm, hyperkeratotic nodule is suggestive of a less cellular, more fibrous lesion (dermatofibroma).

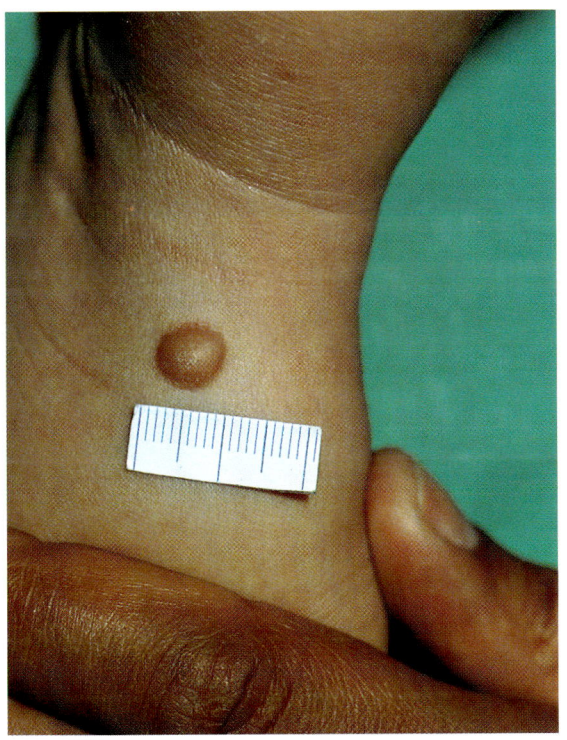

Figure 2.14
Fibrohistiocytoma and dermatofibroma. The pinkish colour of this well-demarcated, smooth, firm nodule is suggestive of a highly cellular lesion (fibrohistiocytoma).

HEMANGIOMAS

Hemangiomas are benign, vascular tumours that appear soon after birth. They are composed of immature capillary vessels situated at various depths in the skin. Differences in clinical presentation are related only to the lesions' extent and depth. Haemangiomas always regress, usually before the first decade of life. They rarely affect the feet.

Strawberry haemangioma (superficial haemangioma, tuberous haemangioma or cherry haemangioma) is a well defined, soft, smooth or lobulated scaly red nodule that reaches a maximum size of a few to many centimetres in diameter within a few months. The lesion is usually warm to the touch and not fully compressible. Resolution is heralded by a softening of the lesions' consistency, the lesions becoming flatter and a modification in their colour – small, pale areas appear in the centre of the lesions.

Deep haemangiomas or cavernous haemangiomas appear as a round or oval, poorly-defined nodule that is characterized by its elastic consistency and is covered with normal-looking skin of a bluish colour. These haemangiomas are less common than superficial forms and tend to resolve more slowly.

Diffuse neonatal haemangiomatosis consists of multiple, cherry-like haemangiomas that are already visible at birth and that are scattered diffusely on the skin. They also involve the visceral organs. Occasionally, lesions may be located on the feet (mainly on the soles). The disorder is often fatal because of complications.

Differential diagnosis

The diagnosis of strawberry haemangiomas is usually straightforward, but differentiated from venous or lymphatic malformations only histologically. Diffuse neonatal haemangiomatosis may mimic congenital self-healing reticulohistiocytosis of Hashimoto–Pritzker, in which the

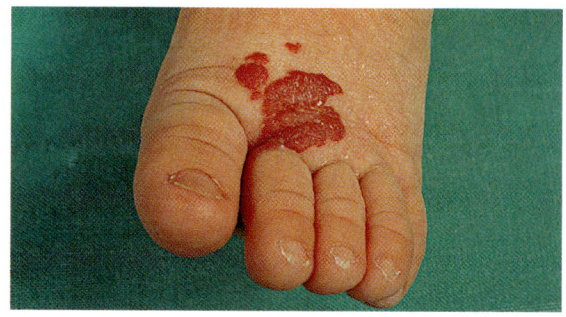
(a)

(b)

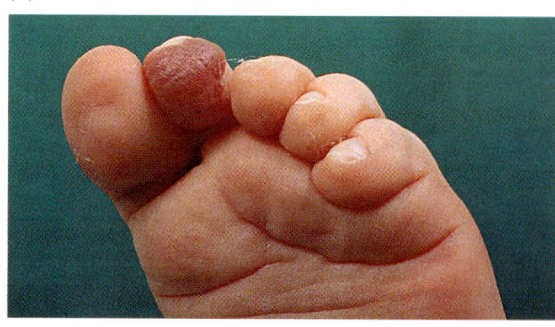
(c)

Figure 2.16(a–c)
Strawberry haemangiomas. They consist of well-defined, soft, smooth, scarlet-red nodules. These lesions in the superficial and mid-dermis are composed of immature capillary vessels (superficial haemangiomas).

lesions are not compressible, presenting frequently with an ulcerated centre and that are, histologically and ultrastructurally, a Langerhans cell histiocytosis.

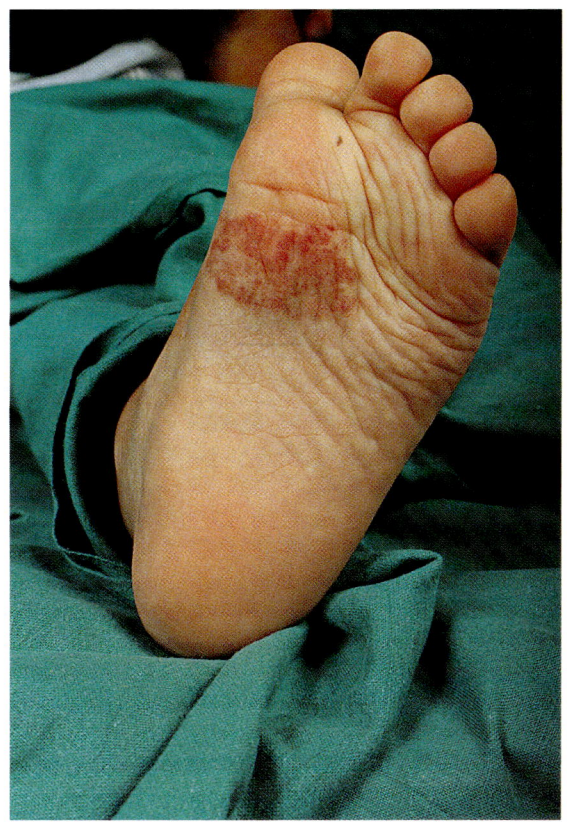

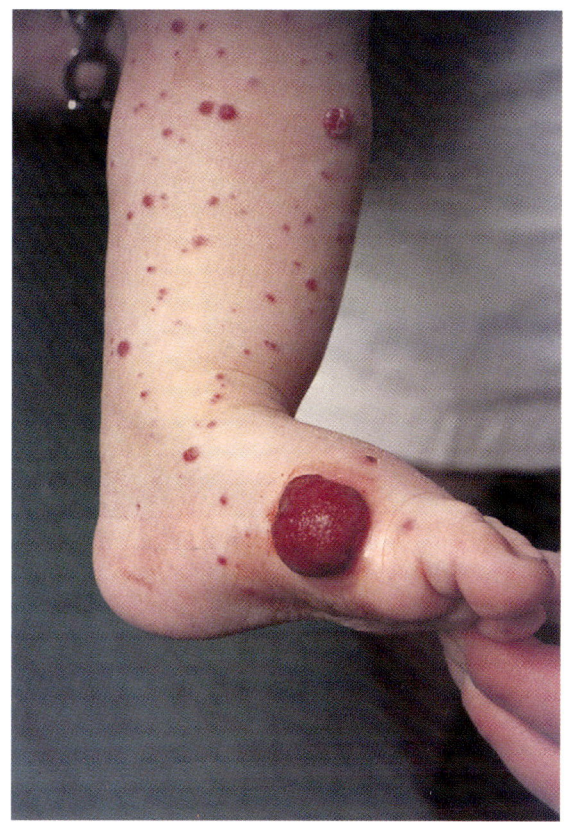

Figure 2.17

Deep haemangiomas. This poorly-defined plaque is characterized by its elasticity and its uneven bluish-red colour.

Figure 2.18

Diffuse neonatal haemangiomatosis. Multiple, cherry-like haemangiomas, present at birth, are suggestive of this disorder.

PORT-WINE STAIN

Port-wine stain (or naevus flammeus) is a congenital vascular malformation of variable size (from a few millimetres to many centimetres) and colour. Pink at the beginning, it turns red or reddish-purple with time. Port-wine stain persists into adulthood and never resolves spontaneously. The lesions are usually unilateral but rarely affect the feet.

In Klippel–Trenaunay–Weber syndrome port-wine stain is associated with deep venous malformations and overgrown soft, bony tissues on the affected limb, which causes an increase in the size of the limb.

Histologically, port-wine stain consists of capillaries and/or venules that are variously distributed in the dermis without the proliferation of endothelial cells. The epidermis is normal.

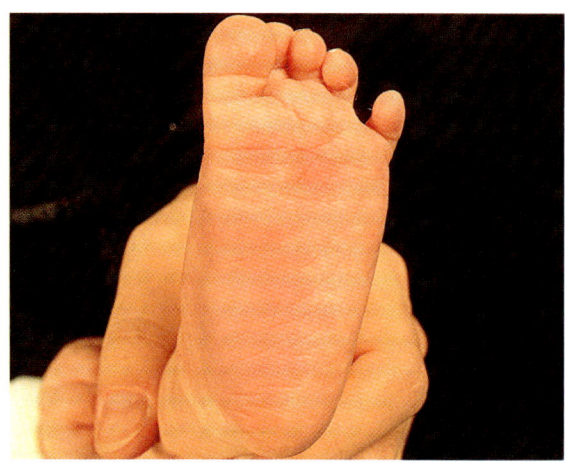

Figure 2.19
Port-wine stain. This congenital, pinkish-red, poorly-defined patch is located unilaterally on the sole.

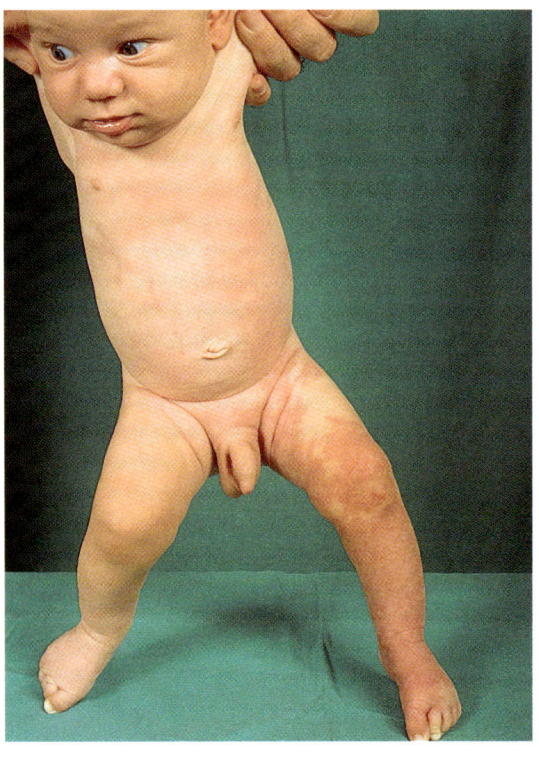

(a)

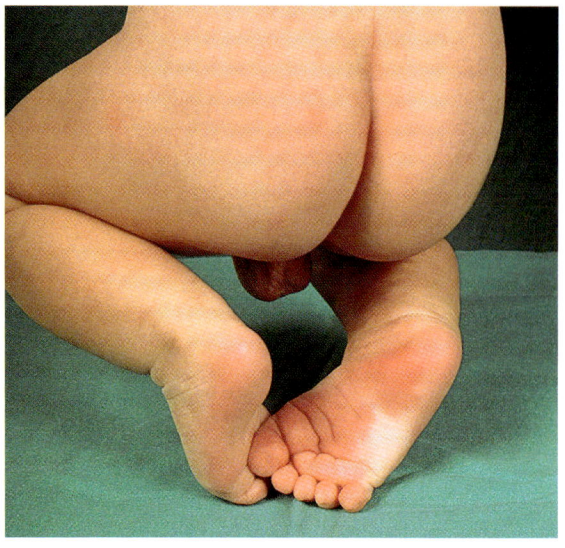

(b)

Figure 2.20(a,b)
Klippel–Trenaunay–Weber syndrome. In this disorder, a port-wine stain on a limb is associated with a deep venous malformation and an increase in the size of the limb involved.

MIBELLI'S ANGIOKERATOMA

Angiokeratomas are skin conditions characterized by a combination of vascular malformation and hyperkeratosis. Two variants of localized angiokeratoma involve the feet: Mibelli's angiokeratoma and angiokeratoma circumscriptum. Histologically, the lesions consist of widely dilated, thin-walled vessels in the upper dermis beneath an area of gross hyperkeratosis.

Clinical features

Mibelli's angiokeratoma consists of dark red, keratotic papules, 2–5 mm in diameter, mainly located over the dorsal and lateral aspects of the toes. Less commonly lesions may be observed on the soles. Although asymptomatic, angiokeratomas bleed easily. The lesions commonly develop during adolescence and are transmitted as an autosomal dominant trait.

Differential diagnosis

Verruca vulgaris is skin coloured and not reddish; its surface is also rougher.

Verrucous haemangioma is a solitary brown to black lesion that is present at birth.

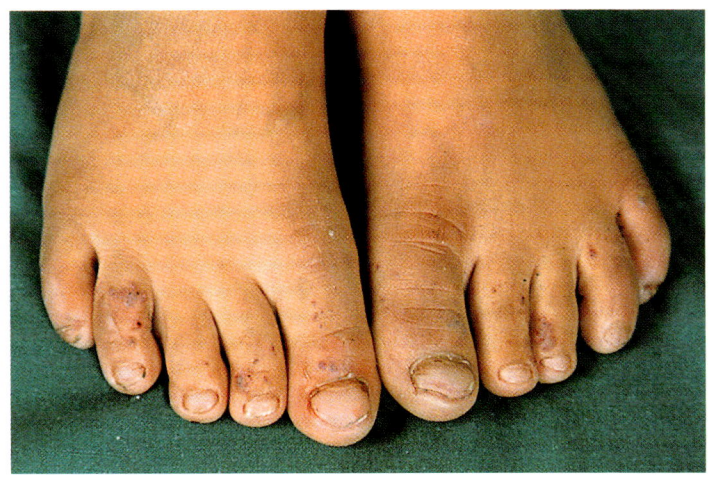

Figure 2.21
Mibelli's angiokeratoma. Discrete, reddish-purple papules are located on the dorsal aspect of toes. Some of these have coalesced into small plaques.

ANGIOKERATOMA CIRCUMSCRIPTUM

Angiokeratoma circumscriptum is usually observed at birth or in early childhood. It presents as a large, solitary, unilateral, linear plaque composed of warty dark red to black papules that have merged together. These lesions tend not to resolve. This malformation may be associated with Klippel–Trenaunay–Weber syndrome.

Differential diagnosis

Angiokeratoma circumscriptum is distinguished from other angiokeratomas and from verrucous haemangioma by virtue of its early onset, its unilateral position and the linear distribution of the plaque, which consists of keratic papules.

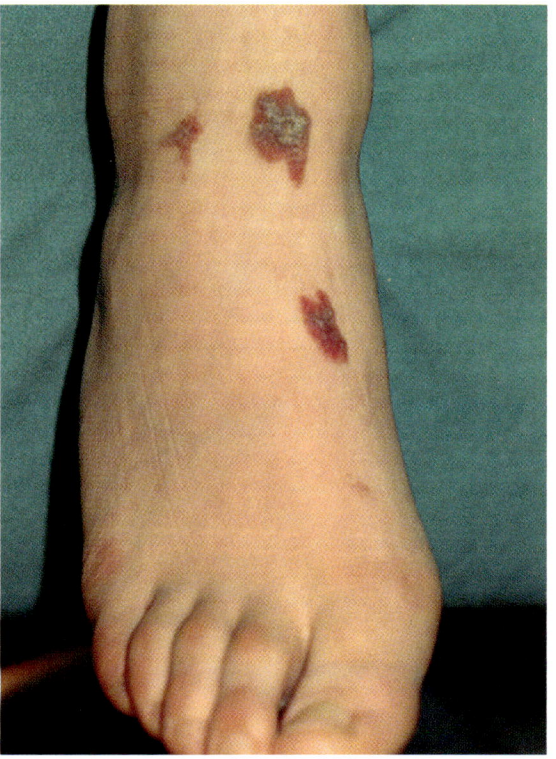

Figure 2.22

Angiokeratoma circumscriptum. These unilateral, irregularly-shaped plaques have scalloped borders and are composed of violaceous to dark red warty papules.

PYOGENIC GRANULOMA

Pyogenic granuloma (PG) is a common vascular tumour that develops after minor trauma. It tends to ulcerate and bleed. The tumour can occur at any age, most frequently on exposed surfaces in children and young adults. In HIV positive patients treated with lamuvidine (for at least 3 months), pyogenic granulomas or paronychia may occur on the toes. The big toe seems to be involved most frequently. Histologically, PG presents with a network of vascular capillary channels with plump endothelial cells in an oedematous stroma.

Clinical features

PG is a solitary, firm, bright red to reddish-brown, pedunculated or sessile tumour that ranges in size from 5 mm to 3 cm. The tumour's base is often surrounded by a collar of acanthotic epidermis. The lesions bleed easily, but are usually painless. The common sites of infection on the feet are the toes and the nail-folds.

Differential diagnosis

Hemangiomas may be ruled out as a result of the tumour's rapid growth, frequent and copious bleeding and its pedunculated appearances.

Glomus tumours are pink or purple, painful nodules.

Molluscum contagiosum is a hemispherical, pink, umbilicated nodule.

Spitz naevus presents as a firm, smooth, nodule in which bleeding and crusting rarely occur.

Amelanotic malignant melanoma requires histopathological examination.

Kaposi's sarcoma is usually multifocal and the collar of acanthotic epidermis is absent. Histologically, the combination of spindle cells and extrarased erythrocytes is diagnostic.

Eccrine poroma may be pedunculated and is erythematous in colour; it rarely bleeds and occurs in patients over 40 years of age. Histopathological examination is necessary.

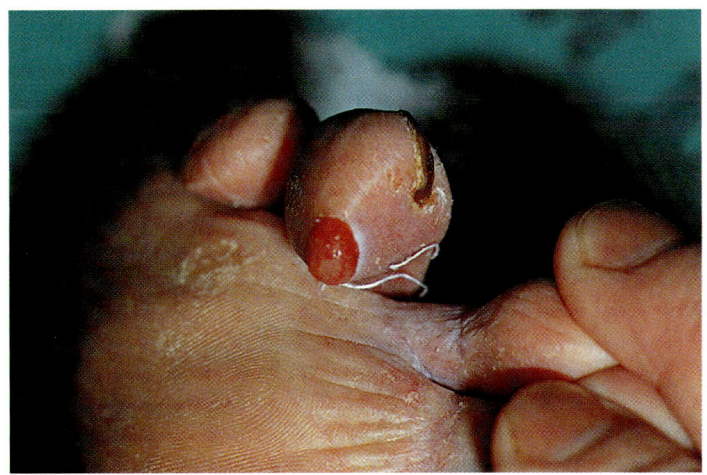

Figure 2.23

Pyogenic granuloma. This is a small, pedunculated, sharply-defined, red, vascular tumour with a history of bleeding. The base of the tumour is surrounded by a whitish epidermal collar.

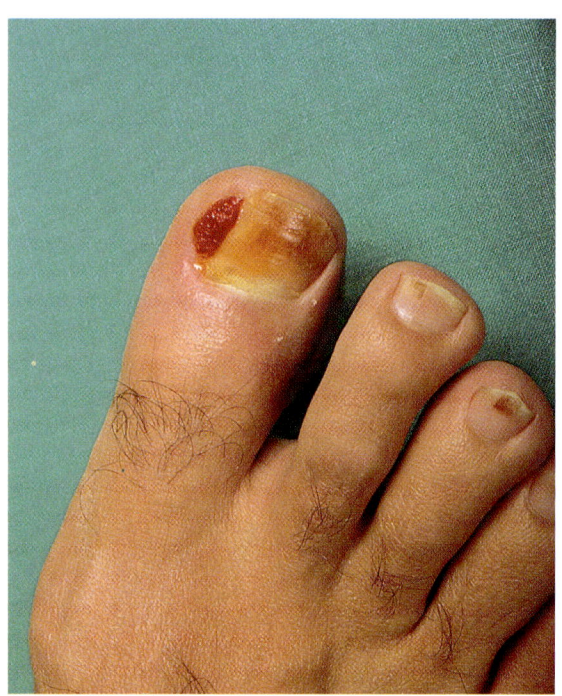

Figure 2.24(a,b)

Pyogenic granuloma. The big toes of these HIV positive patients treated with lamuvidine have developed vascular tumours along the borders of the nail-plates.

(a)

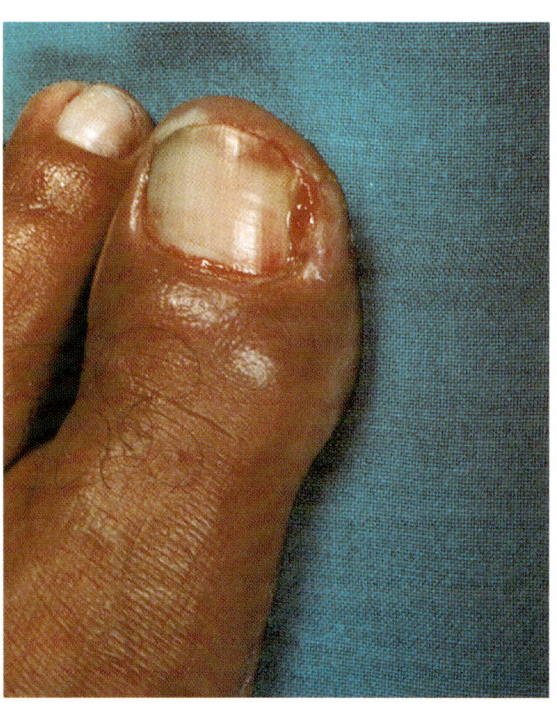

(b)

BLUE RUBBER-BLEB NAEVI SYNDROME

Blue rubber-bleb naevi syndrome is a peculiar angiomatosis characterized by numerous cavernous haemangiomas that involve the skin, mucous membranes and frequently the viscera. The lesions typically consist of numerous, painful, soft, blue nodules scattered randomly on the trunk and limbs. These lesions are easily compressible and refill promptly when pressure is removed. The syndrome is often detected at birth or in early infancy and is persistent. Histologically the lesions consist of very widely dilated vein-like structures in the dermis and subcutaneous fat, some of which may thrombose and organize.

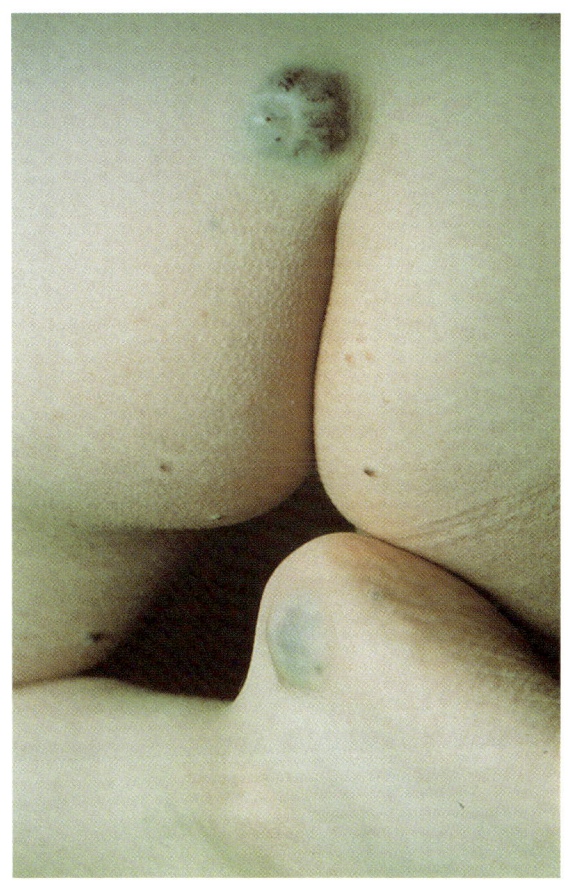

Clinical features

Tender, painful, blue, nipple-like nodules of a rubbery consistency may be observed on the soles. Hyperidrosis is often apparent on the surface of the lesions.

Figure 2.25
Blue-rubber naevi syndrome. These two soft, blue nodules are painful, easily compressible and refill promptly when pressure is removed.

Differential diagnosis

The typical painful, blue, rubbery, nipple-like lesions allow easy differentiation from other vascular malformations and glomangioma.

KAPOSI'S SARCOMA

Kaposi's sarcoma (KS) is a systemic vascular tumour that has four distinct subsets. Classic KS mainly affects elderly, male patients of Mediterranean or Jewish extraction, predominantly involving the lower legs and feet. Its course is indolent and chronic. Endemic KS occurs in African children and young adults involving lymph nodes, bone and skin. Iatrogenic immunosuppressive drug-associated KS occurs in kidney transplant patients. Its clinical course is similar to classic KS, although it is more aggressive. Epidemic, HIV-associated KS occurs mainly in homosexual males with AIDS and has a rapidly progressive course that involves the skin, mucous membranes, lymph nodes and viscera. Skin lesions are widespread but appear most often on the lower extremities, trunk and head.

Histopathologically, a fully-developed KS lesion is characterized by interweaving bands of spindle cells and vascular structures lined with atypical endothelial cells that are embedded in a network of reticular and collagen fibres. Extravasated erythrocytes with haemosiderin deposition are also present.

Clinical features

Cutaneous KS lesions most often start as pink to bluish-red asymptomatic macules. These evolve into firm papules and nodules that sometimes have a hyperkeratotic or verrucous surface. The lesions progress slowly and may coalesce to form large plaques. Lesions occasionally ulcerate and they bleed easily. They may be associated with oedema of the involved foot or leg. Large lesions of the sole may impede the ability to walk.

Differential diagnosis

Many tumours must be considered in the differential diagnosis of fully-developed KS lesions.

Pyogenic granuloma is usually solitary and surrounded by a collar of acanthotic epidermis. It develops rapidly after trauma and bleeds easily.

Verrucous haemangioma is a solitary brown to black lesion that is present at birth.

Glomus tumours are painful.

Histiocytomas are firm and yellow-brown in colour.

Malignant melanoma may be ruled out by epiluminescence and histology.

Eccrine poroma is a solitary, moist, pink nodule. In all these tumours, confirmatory skin biopsies should always be undertaken.

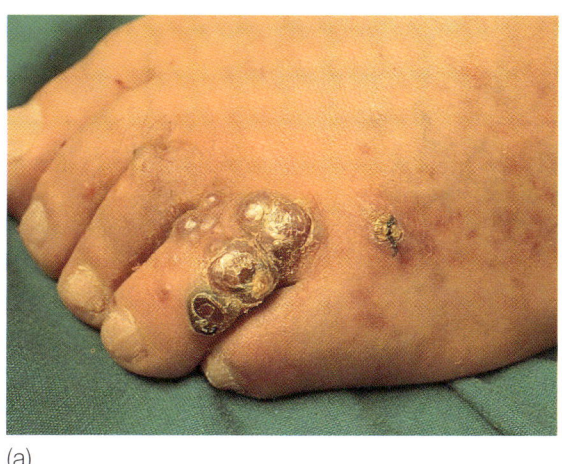

(a)

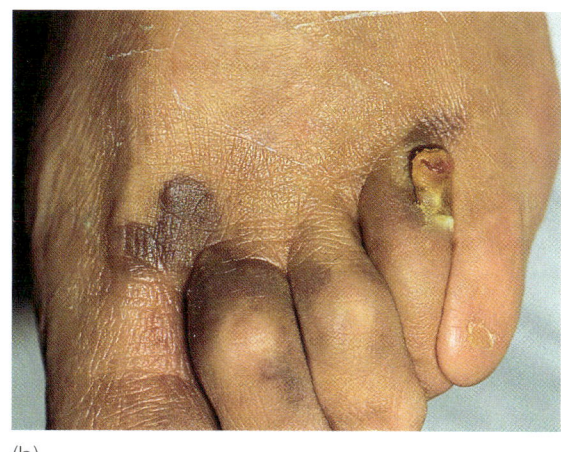

(b)

Figure 2.26(a,b)
Classic Kaposi's sarcoma. Bluish-red asymptomatic nodules on the dorsal aspect of the toes.

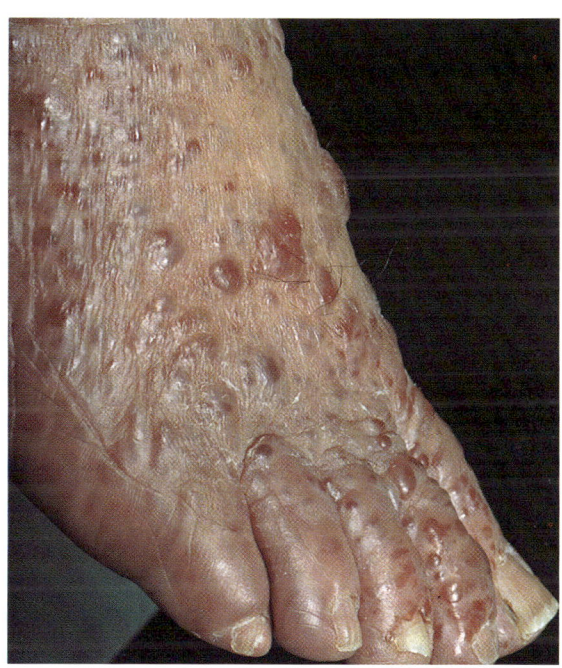

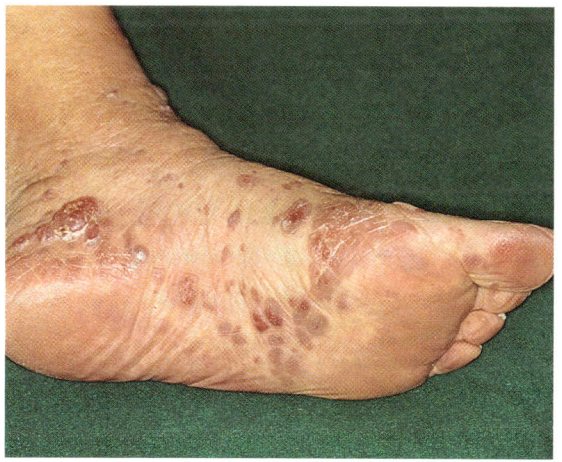

Figure 2.27
Classic Kaposi's sarcoma. On the back of this foot, the lesions have slowly coalesced to form a large plaque.

Figure 2.28
Classic Kaposi's sarcoma. The nodular lesions and plaque may extend to the soles and hence may impede the ability to walk. (Photograph courtesy of Professor Aldo Finzi.)

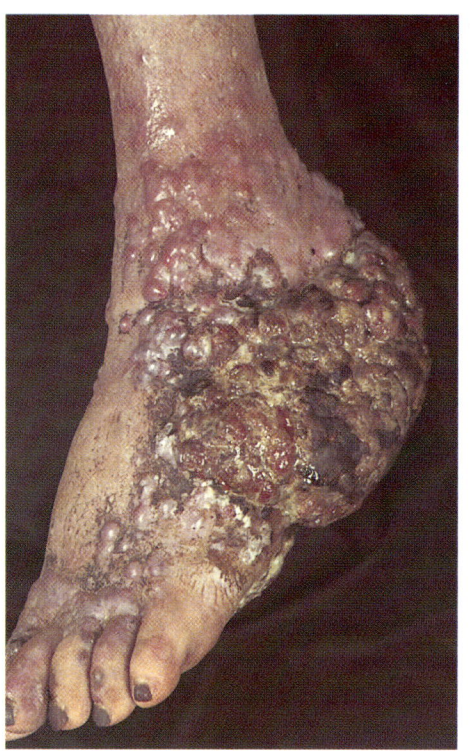

← **Figure 2.29**

Classic Kaposi's sarcoma. In this patient, the nodular lesions merged into a large, vegetating, ulcerated, plaque with a tendency to bleed.

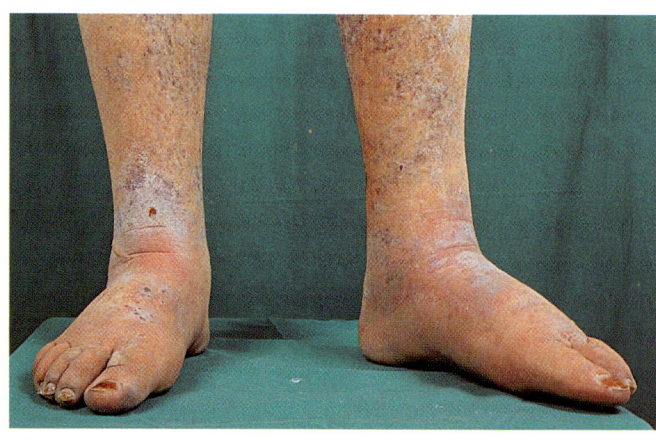

↑
Figure 2.30

Classic Kaposi's sarcoma. The feet frequently become oedematous.

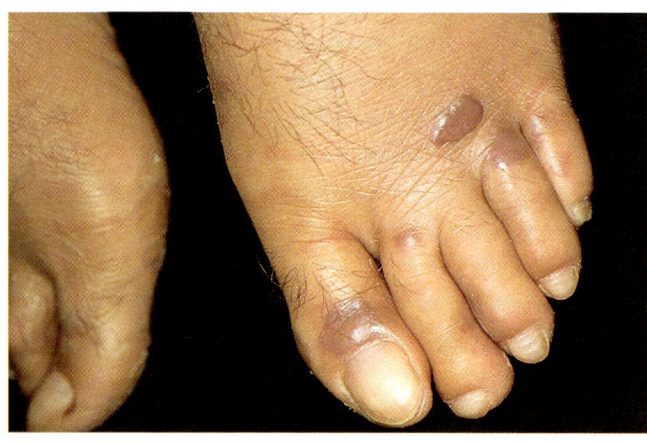

(a)

Figure 2.31(a,b)

Epidemic HIV-associated Kaposi's sarcoma. In these patients the nodular lesions have assumed a lance-like shape and are progressing rapidly.

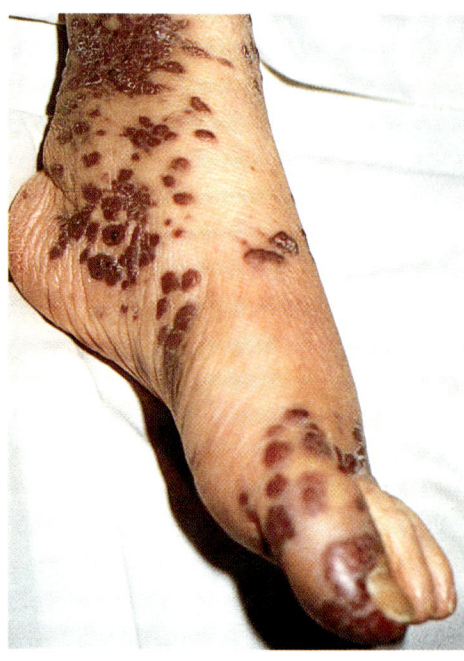

(b)

BLUEFARB–STEWART SYNDROME

Bluefarb–Stewart syndrome consists of cutaneous lesions that arise on a limb as a consequence of an underlying arteriovenous malformation. These lesions resemble Kaposi's sarcoma. The lesions start during the first or second decade of life and involve the lower extremities unilaterally. Histopathologically, the entire dermis is occupied by an arteriovenous shunt. This consists of a markedly increased number of thick-walled blood vessels lined with plump endothelial cells in association with extravasated erythrocytes and numerous syderophages.

Clinical features

The lesion begins as violaceous macules or patches that develop into soft, smooth, non-tender reddish to purplish papules or nodules. In some cases the cutaneous nodules are painful and become ulcerated. Sites of predilection are the first three toes of the foot and the dorsal aspect of the foot. A sensation of increased warmth and a palpable thrill are the result of the underlying arteriovenous malformation.

Differential diagnosis

Kaposi's sarcoma is ruled out by the presence of the underlying arteriovenous malformation, which is readily demonstrated through sections stained with haematoxylineosin.

Pyogenic granuloma is a solitary lesion with a collar of acanthotic epidermis.

Gougerot and Blum disease (pigmented purpuric lichenoid dermatosis) consists of clusters of violaceous lichenoid papules.

Klippel–Trenaunay–Weber syndrome is characterized by congenital haemangiomas and soft tissue hypertrophy.

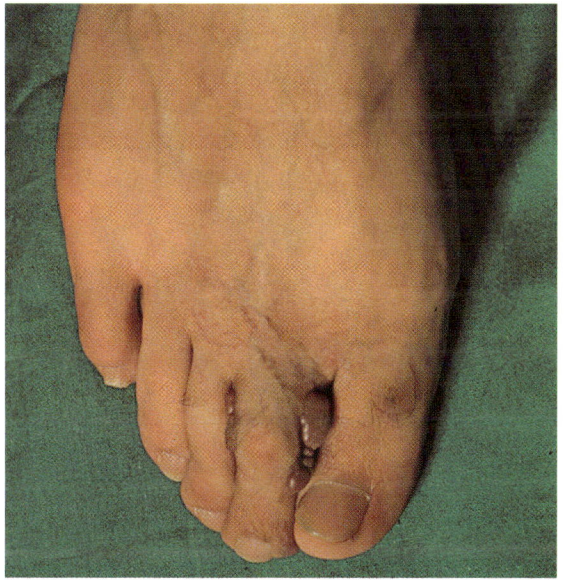

Figure 2.32(a)

Bluefarb–Stewart syndrome. This condition is characterized by cutaneous lesions that resemble Kaposi's sarcoma as a consequence of the underlying arterio-venous malformation. Sites of predilection are the dorsal aspect of the foot (a) and the first three toes (b and c). A sensation of increased warmth and, occasionally, a palpable thrill are indicative of the underlying malformation. (Photograph courtesy of Professor Elvio Alessi.)

(continued on the next page)

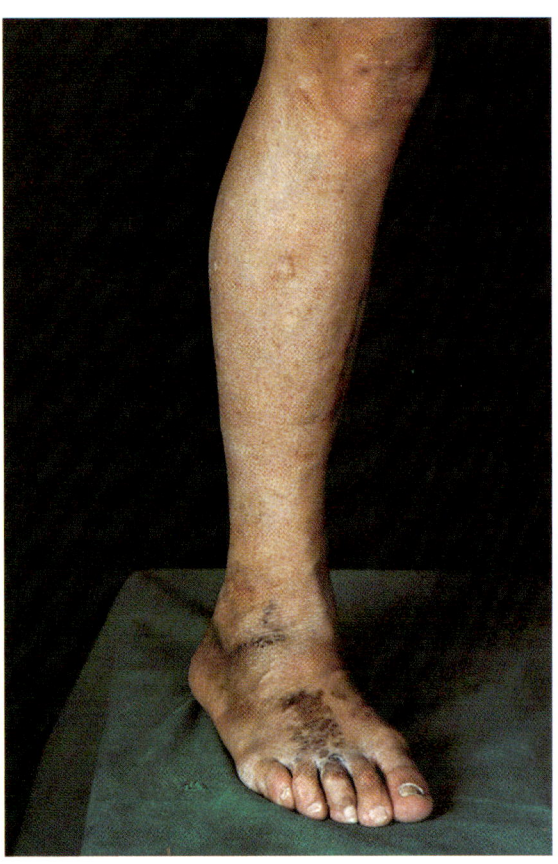

Figure 2.32(b)
Bluefarb–Stewart syndrome.

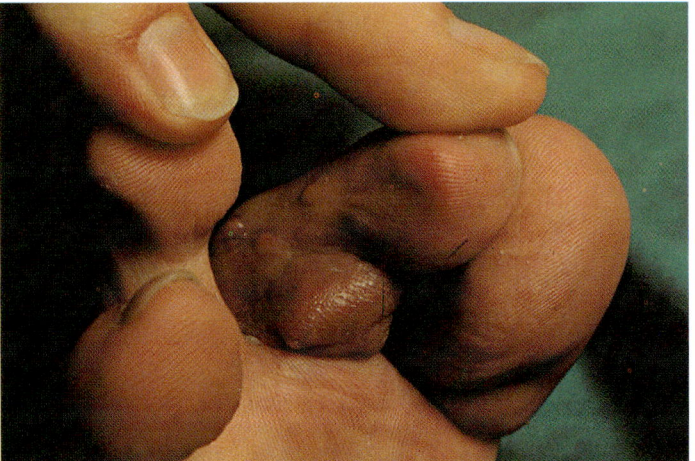

Figure 2.32(c)
Bluefarb–Stewart syndrome.

LYMPHANGIOMA CIRCUMSCRIPTUM

Lymphangioma circumscriptum is the most common type of lymphangioma. It consists of a large number of thin-walled vesicles that are either isolated or grouped into a plaque. The disorder is usually asymptomatic and may involve virtually any area of the skin but it is rarely found on the feet. It most commonly occurs at birth, the majority of the tumours having appeared by the age of 5 years. On pathological examination the lesion is seen to consist of numerous extremely thin-walled lymphatic channels with only one layer of lining endothelium cells on the superficial dermis.

Clinical features

Lymphangioma circumscriptum manifests as multiple small vesicles, white to purple in colour, that resemble frog spawn. The purple colour is due to the presence of blood. The lesions are ruptured easily by friction, but new lesions develop fairly rapidly.

Differential diagnosis

Mibelli's angiokeratoma is characterized by dark-red, isolated keratic papules, mainly located on the dorsal aspect of the toes.

Angiokeratoma circumscriptum is a plaque composed of warty, dark-red papules.

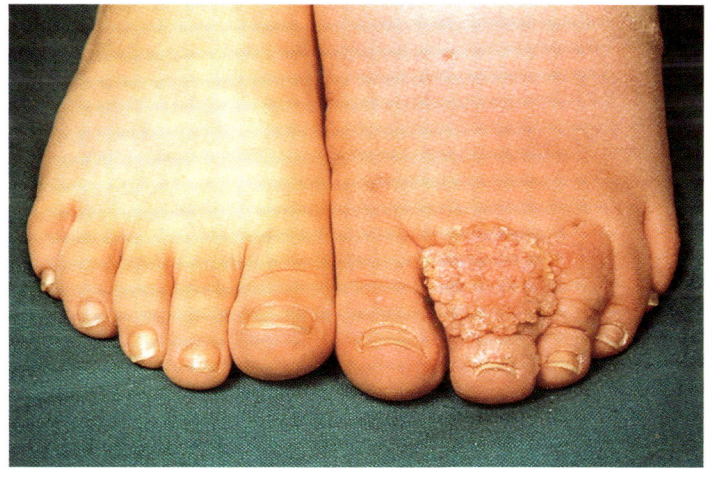

Figure 2.33

Lymphangioma circumscriptum. A cluster of wart-like papular vesicles is located on a toe. Each papular vesicle represents a widely dilated, lymph-containing lymphatic in the uppermost part of the dermis. These lesions have been compared in appearance to frog spawn.

ECCRINE POROMA

Eccrine poroma is a solitary, asymptomatic, benign, pink to red tumour with a sessile or broadly pedunculated base. The lesion is well defined and may be surrounded by a gutter-like depression. It can attain 1–2 cm in diameter. Ulceration may occasionally occur but only in tumours situated at points of pressure. The great majority of lesions are found on the soles of patients who have passed the age of 40 years. The histologic aspect is distinctive. This consists of broad, anastomosing strands of uniform, small, cuboidal cells with basophilic round nuclei and moderate amounts of pale, strongly PAS-positive cytoplasm.

Differential diagnosis

Pyogenic granuloma usually develops rapidly after trauma. It is surrounded by a collar of acanthotic epidermis and bleeds easily.

Malignant melanoma may be ruled out by epiluminescence, but histologic examination will also be necessary.

Verrucous haemangioma is a lesion that is present at birth.

Kaposi's sarcoma is usually multifocal.

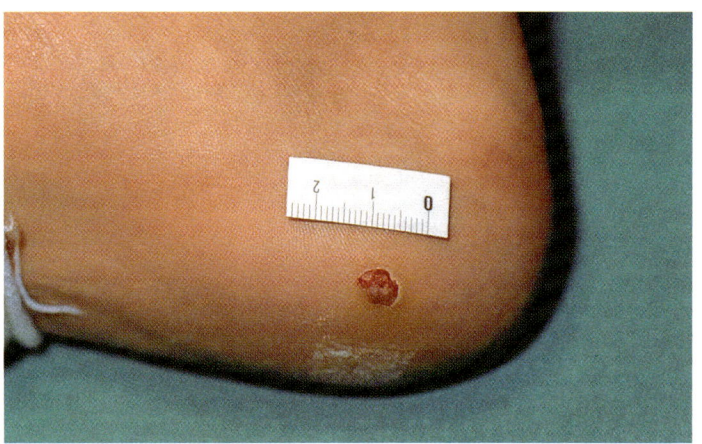

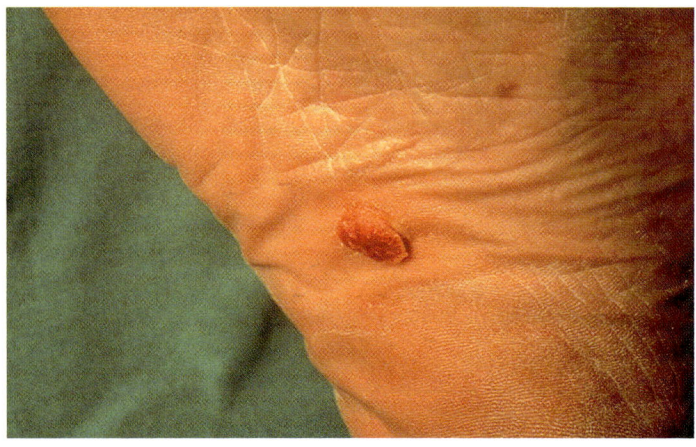

Figure 2.34(a–c)
Eccrine poroma. The vast majority of these solitary, asymptomatic lesions occur on the soles in the form of well defined, red tumours, frequently with a pedunculated base (b and c). They may attain a diameter of more than 2 cm (c).

(a)

(b)

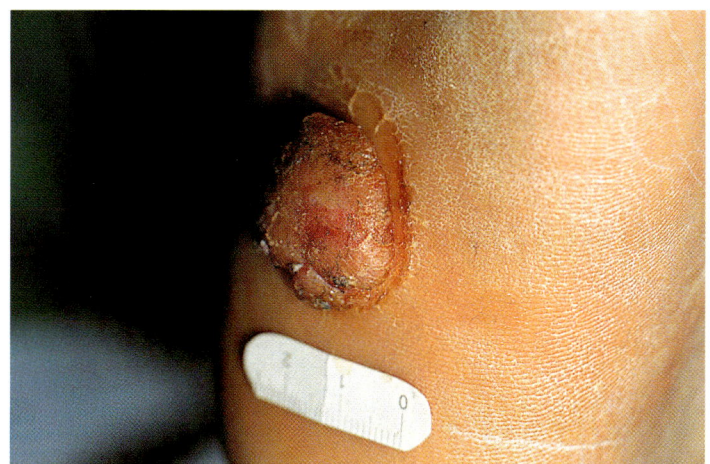

(c)

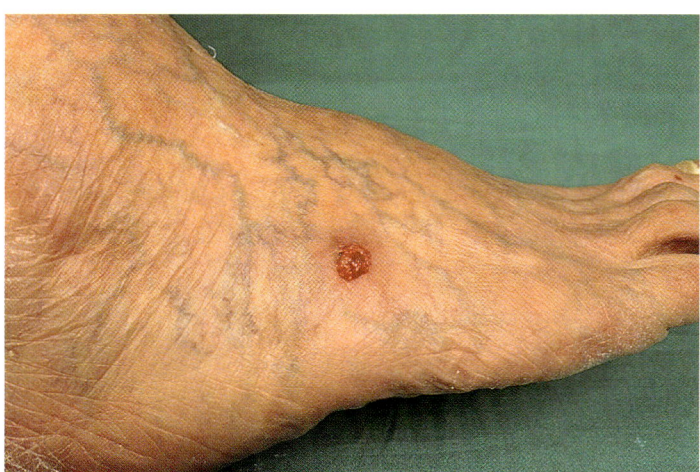

Figure 2.35

Eccrine poroma. A tumour on the back of the foot is rare. In this example the lesions mimic a pyogenic granuloma.

BOWEN'S DISEASE

Bowen's disease is an intra-epidermal carcinoma that appears as an isolated, well-demarcated, scaly, sometimes hyperkeratotic or crusted, red, irregular plaque. The lesion is slightly raised and tends to enlarge gradually. Ulceration is a sign of invasive growth. Bowen's disease may occur anywhere, but typically on the lower leg in females. However, it is rare on the feet, mainly involving the dorsal aspect.

Differential diagnosis

Psoriasis is rare as an isolated plaque. Auspitz's sign (small points of bleeding after removal of scales) may be induced.

Eczematous dermatitis is pruriginous, disappearing readily when steroids are applied.

Superficial basal cell carcinoma presents with a characteristic, raised, rolled edge.

Solar keratosis is rare on the feet. Histopathological examination is required.

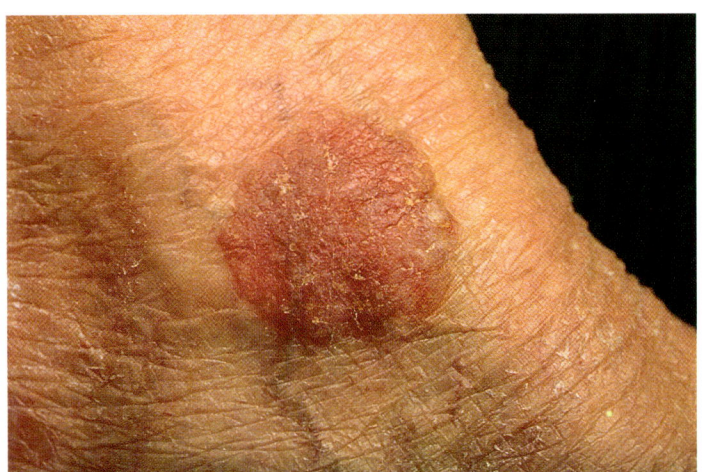

Figure 2.36
Bowen's disease. This isolated lesion is well demarcated, slightly raised, reddish brown and scaling.

KERATOACANTHOMA

Keratoacanthoma is a relatively common, rapidly growing, self-limiting, benign epidermal tumour. The fully-developed tumour consists of a rounded, firm, flesh-coloured nodule. This is crater-like in shape and has a central keratinous plug. Its diameter varies from one to a few centimetres. The surrounding skin is undamaged. Spontaneous healing takes a few months and this is characterized by the shedding of the horny plug. Keratoacanthomas most often occur as solitary lesions on areas of patients over the age of 40 years that have been exposed to the sun. The feet are very rarely affected (on the dorsal aspect), while the soles are always spared. In cases of multiple tumours (multiple self-limiting epithelioma of Ferguson–Smith or generalized eruptive keratoacanthoma of Gryzbowski), lesions occur more readily on the backs of the feet. Histopathologically the lesions are characterized by the keratinous plug, pseudo-epitheliomatous hyperplasia, overhanging epidermal margins near the keratinous plug, relative lack of cellular abnormalities and inflammatory cell infiltrate at the base of the lesion.

Differential diagnosis

Squamous cell carcinoma lacks the regular, crater-like shape and the central plug. It also has an older age of onset.

Viral warts are irregular, vegetating and not crater-like in shape.

Eccrine poroma is a well-demarcated, firm, red lesion with a smooth surface which mainly involves the soles.

Fibrohistiocytoma is a hard lesion that feels like a small button.

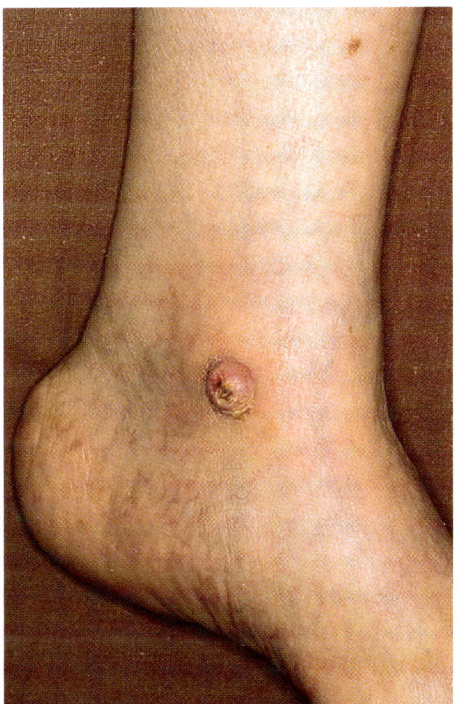

Figure 2.37

Keratoacanthoma. This round, firm, flesh-coloured, crater-shaped nodule has lost its central horny plug. This is a sign of spontaneous resolution. (Photograph courtesy of Professor Aldo Finzi.)

SQUAMOUS CELL CARCINOMA

Squamous cell carcinoma (SCC) is a malignant proliferation of keratinocytes that presents as a firm, indurated, expanding, sometimes ulcerated mass. The most common sites for SCCs are sun-exposed areas of the body, and tumours frequently arise on pre-existing skin lesions. The lower limbs are the most frequent site for this tumour in black Africans and in natives of tropical countries. Metastases to regional lymph nodes tend to be associated with the larger and deeper SCCs. SCC is rare under the age of 40 years; however, incidence of the disease increases with age. Histopathologically, SCC consists of malignant epidermal cells that extend beyond the dermo-epidermal junction into the dermis. The invading cells show different degrees of differentiation and keratinization. Well-differentiated tumours (as in carcinoma cuniculatum) have areas of progressive keratinization (horny pearls), while in highly-malignant tumours the cells are atypical, mitotic figures are frequent and keratinization is almost absent.

Clinical features

Carcinoma cuniculatum is a typical variant of SCC that involves the feet. It presents as slow-growing, painful, exophytic, fungating masses of long duration. Sinus tracts open on to the surface of the skin. Foul-smelling, greasy material can be expressed from the sinuses when pressure is applied. The most common areas of infection are the ball of the sole (53%), the toes (21%), the heel (16%) and, occasionally, the mid-plantar region and dorsal aspect of the foot. Metastases are very rare.

Differential diagnosis

The clinical aspect and the site of involvement on the foot are typical of carcinoma cuniculatum.

Masses of viral warts are less vegetating and do not have sinus tract openings.

Deep mycoses and verrucous tuberculosis (TBC) are easily ruled out by cultures and by their good response to treatment.

Acrolentiginous melanoma is not a cauliflower-like shaped tumour and it is usually pigmented.

Eccrine poroma is a solitary, often sessile, well demarcated, firm, red lesion with a smooth or lobulated surface.

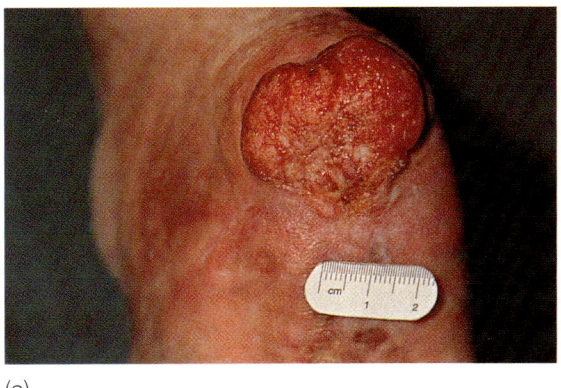
(a)

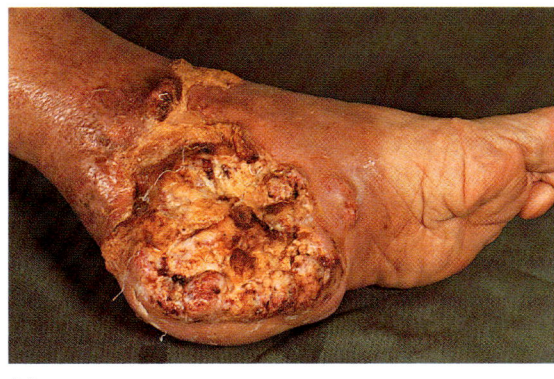
(b)

Figure 2.38(a,b)

Carcinoma cuniculatum. This is the most common form of SCC to involve the feet. It presents as exophytic, fungating masses. In long-standing lesions the openings of the sinus tracts are readily observed. The heel is involved in 16% of cases.

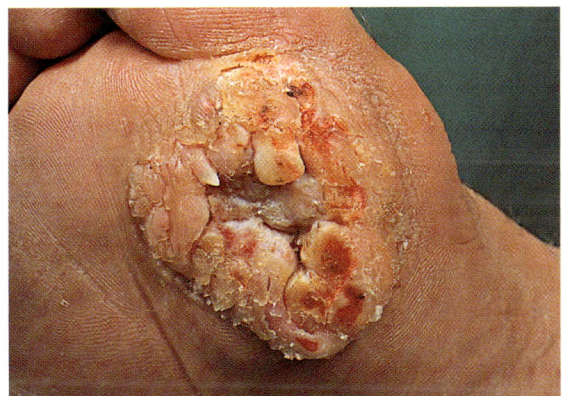
(a)

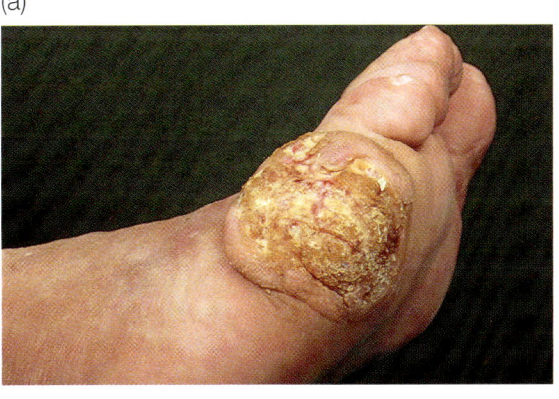
(b)

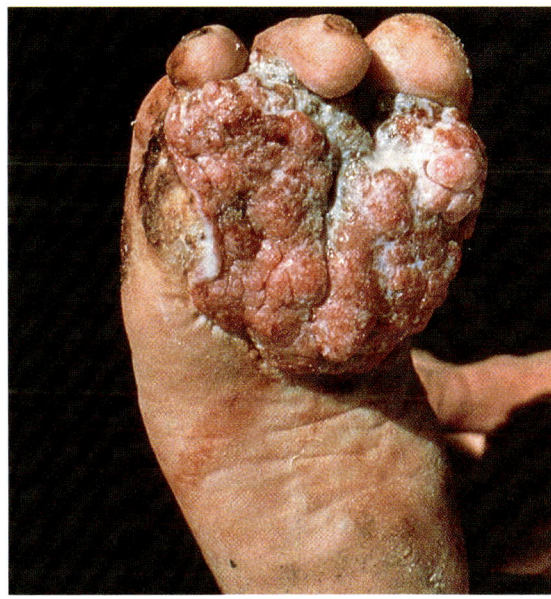
(c)

Figure 2.39(a–c)

Carcinoma cuniculatum. The ball of the soles is the most common site of involvement (53%). The expanding mass in (c) is covered with a foul-smelling, greasy material that has issued from the sinuses.

NAEVOID BASAL-CELL CARCINOMA SYNDROME

Naevoid basal-cell carcinoma syndrome is an autosomal dominant condition characterized by numerous basal-cell carcinomas, pits on the palms and soles, jaw cysts, skeletal anomalies, ectopic calcifications, ophthalmic defects and a facial appearance typical of the condition. The characteristic facial appearance is a broad nasal root, frontal bosselations, well developed supraorbital ridges, hypertelorism and mild mandibular prognathism.

The skin lesions may appear at puberty, but palmoplantar pits may be noted as early as the second year of life. Histologically, the pits are incipient basal-cell carcinomas, above which are attenuated zones of cornification.

Patients with this syndrome continue to develop basal-cell carcinomas with increasing frequency throughout their lives.

Clinical features

The typical features on feet are circular-shaped pits, 1–3 mm in diameter, occasionally surrounded by a thin rim of erythema. There may be only a few or hundreds of these pits. They are usually more numerous on the lateral surfaces of the soles. Plantar pits are more common in adults than in children.

Differential diagnosis

The diagnosis of naevoid basal-cell carcinoma syndrome is relatively easy because of its highly distinctive symptoms.

The plantar pits of Darier's disease are usually associated with lesions on seborrhoeic areas and on the nails. Punctate keratoderma is characterized by yellowish-brown, round, keratotic papules with central keratotic plugs. Histopathology will confirm diagnosis.

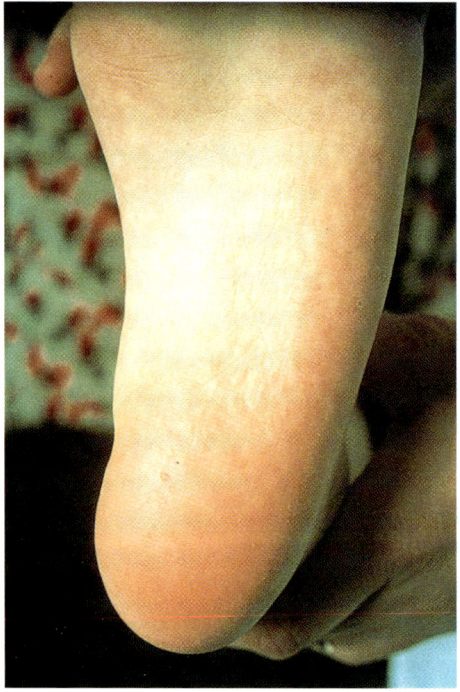

Figure 2.40

Naevoid basal-cell carcinoma syndrome. Only a few pits are present on the sole of this patient.

CONGENITAL MELANOCYTIC NAEVI

Congenital melanocytic naevi are proliferations of melanocytes that are present at birth. These naevi can be divided into small (less than 1.5 cm), intermediate (less than 20 cm) and giant (with a diameter greater than 20 cm) naevi. The vast majority of congenital naevi are small, and about 1% of babies present with this type of naevi at birth. A classic congenital naevus consists pathologically of melanocytes situated in the reticular dermis. Both angiocentricity and adnexocentricity of the melanocytes are typical.

Clinical features

The vast majority of congenital naevi on the feet are small. These are round or oval, smooth, sharply-demarcated macules or plaques of varying colour from brown to black. The lesions are usually devoid of hairs, grow slowly and frequently darken with age.

Differential diagnosis

Lentigines in Peutz–Jeghers syndrome are smooth, brown, macular lesions mainly located in the buccal mucosa and centrofacial area. These lesions are associated with gastrointestinal polyps.

Large, acquired Clark's naevi (dysplastic naevi) are usually not as dark as small congenital naevi, but histological examination is necessary to confirm the diagnosis.

Vascular abnormalities are easily differentiated with epiluminescence.

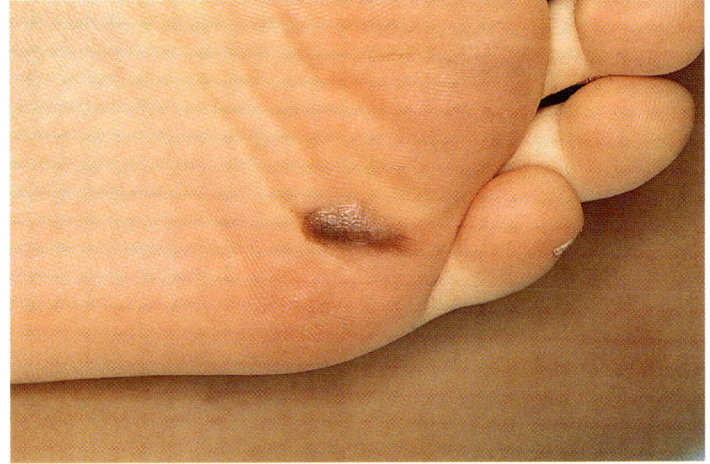

Figure 2.41(a)
Small congenital melanocytic naevi. In this example, there are two oval, smooth, sharply-demarcated, brown plaques that are devoid of hair.

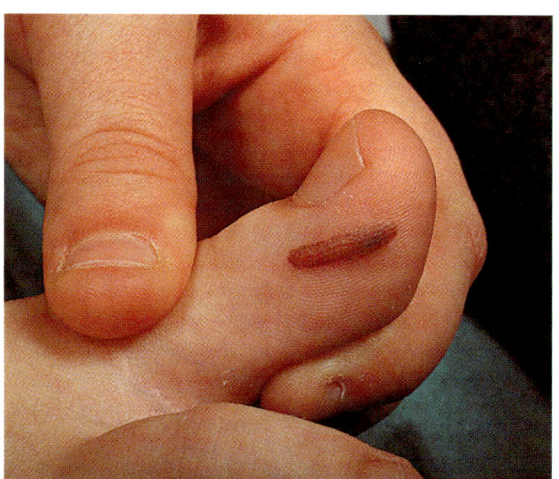

Figure 2.41(b)
Small congenital melanocytic naevi.

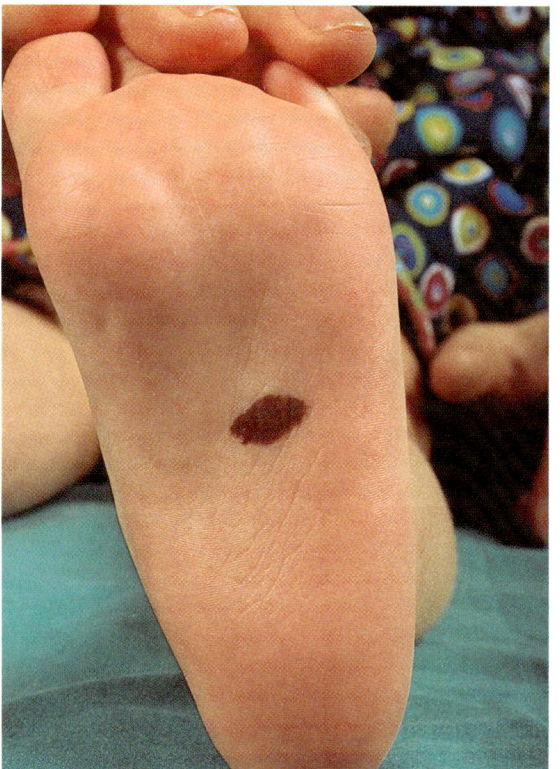

Figure 2.42
Intermediate congenital melanocytic naevus.
This black, oval lesion has a diameter of more
than 1.5 cm.

ACQUIRED MELANOCYTIC NAEVI

Acquired melanocytic naevi are clusters of melanocytic naevus cells that derive from epidermal melanocytes or dermal melanocytes after birth. The most frequent melanocytic naevi that arise from epidermal melanocytes are junctional naevi, compound naevi, intradermal naevi and dysplastic naevi (these four types are also called Clark's naevi) and Spitz naevi.

The most frequent variants of naevi that derive from dermal melanocytes and that are seen on the feet are the common and the cellular blue naevi.

Pigmented lesions on the feet are common. Pigmented naevi can be observed on the soles in about 8% of white patients and in about 20% of black patients. These often appear during childhood and tend to increase in size and number during puberty.

Clinical features: Junctional naevi

Clinical

Junctional naevi present as sandy-brown, poorly-defined, round or oval macules less than 1 cm in diameter. This type of naevi is seen most frequently on the palms and on the soles.

Histopathological

Nests of melanocytes will be observed at the dermo-epidermal junction.

Differential diagnosis

Lentigines in Peutz–Jegher's syndrome may be present on the feet but is more usually associated with pigmented lesions in the buccal mucosa and with gastrointestinal polyps.

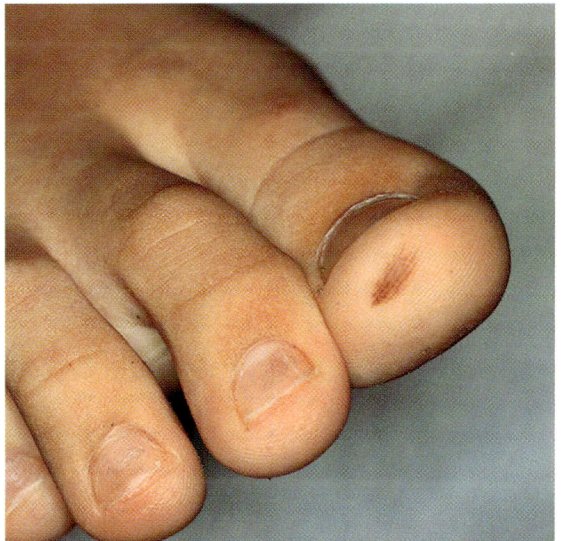

Figure 2.43(a)
Junctional naevi. Junctional naevi are round or oval, poorly-defined, brown macules less than 1 cm in diameter.

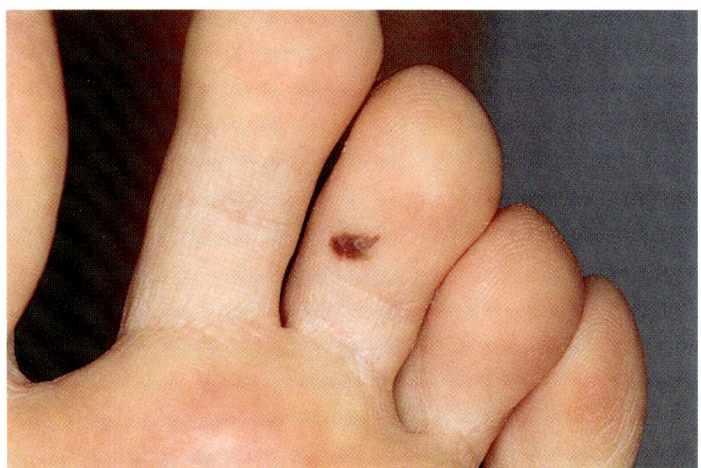

Figure 2.43(b)
Junctional naevi.

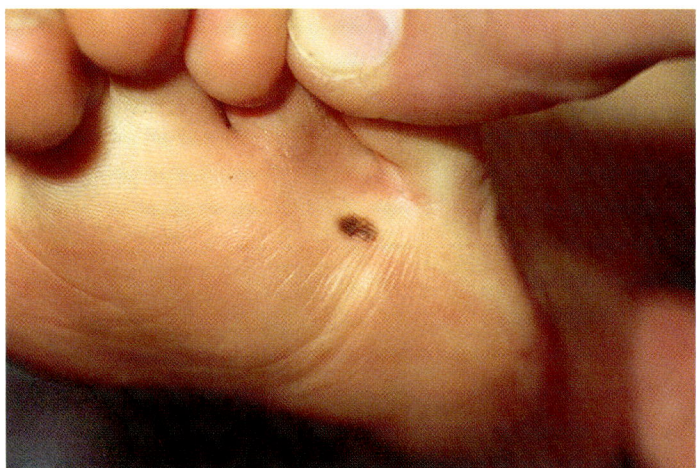

Figure 2.43(c)
Junctional naevi.

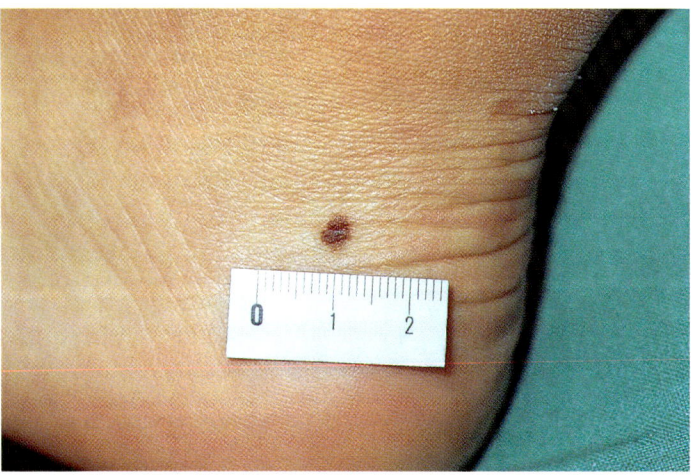

Figure 2.43(d)
Junctional naevi.

Clinical features: Compound naevi

Clinical

Compound naevi are the more usual form of acquired naevi found in young adults. These are sharply circumscribed, round or oval and 3–6 mm in diameter; they vary in colour from a light tan to dark–brown. These naevi may be slightly raised or papillomatous on the dorsal aspect of the feet but are smooth and flat on the soles.

Histopathological

Nests of melanocytes will be observed at the dermo-epidermal junction, and clusters of melanocytes within the papillary dermis.

Differential diagnosis

Small congenital naevi are usually darker than acquired compound naevi, but histopathology is necessary to distinguish between the two. Pigmented basal cell carcinoma of the dorsal aspect of the foot is opalescent and telangiectatic.

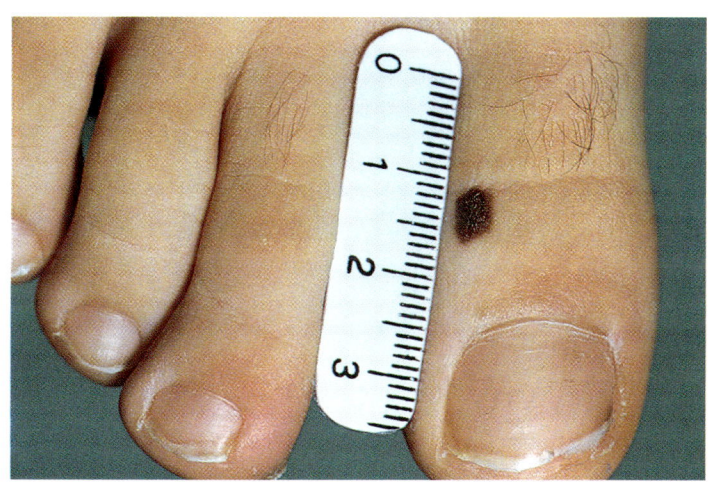

Figure 2.44(a)

Compound naevi. Compound naevi are sharply demarcated, round or oval, pigmented lesions that vary in colour from light tan to dark brown. These are the most common form of acquired naevi observed in young adults and, on the dorsal aspect of the feet or toes, may be slightly raised or papillomatous.

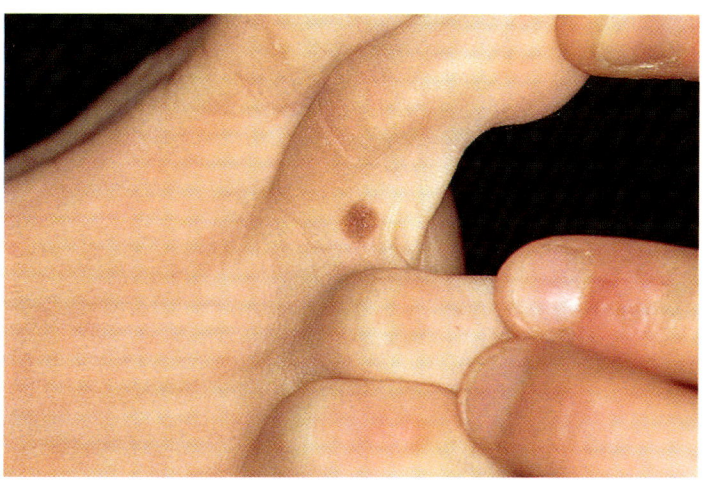

Figure 2.44(b)

Compound naevi.

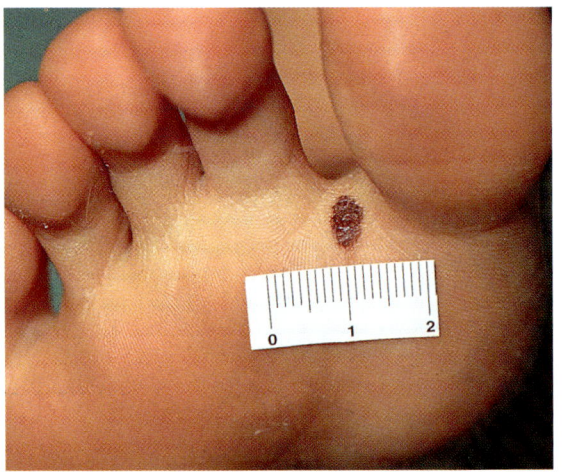

Figure 2.44(c)
Compound naevi.

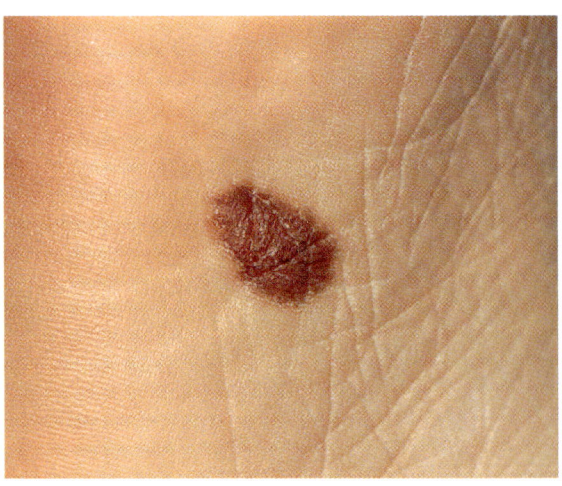

Figure 2.44(d)
Compound naevi.

Clinical features: Intradermal naevi

Clinical

Intradermal naevi appear after adolescence and present as smooth, dome-shaped flesh-coloured nodules. These are found on the feet.

Histopathological

Nests of melanocytes will be observed in a thickened papillary dermis.

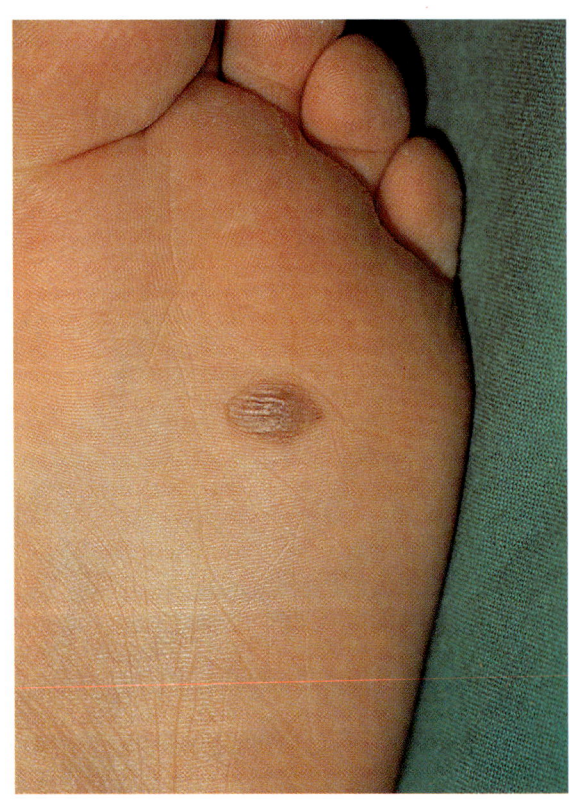

Figure 2.45
Intradermal naevus. This naevus presents as a well-demarcated, skin-coloured to light-brown lesion. These naevi rarely occur on the feet.

Clinical features: Dyplastic naevi

Clinical

Dysplastic naevi are large (more than 6 mm), asymmetrical, irregularly- or poorly-demarcated lesions with an irregular pigmentation that varies from various shades of brown to black. They may arise sporadically or may display a familial pattern. When located on the plantar surface, this type of naevus has been designated as 'acral lentiginous naevi'.

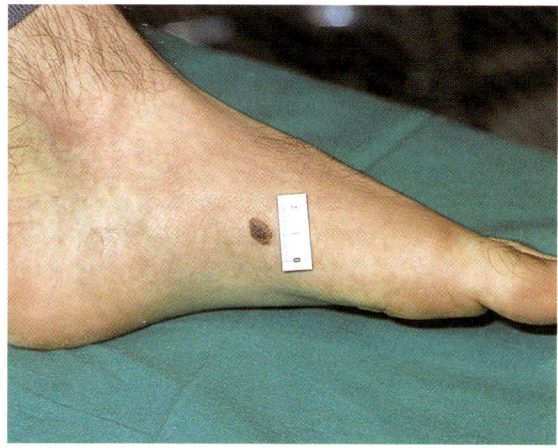

(a)

Histopathological

The great majority of dysplastic naevi are compound naevi with architectural and cytological abnormalities. Architectural abnormalities include the large size of the lesion, lentiginous melanocytic hyperplasia of melanocytes in the basal layer and the focal elongation of epidermal rete ridges. Cytological abnormalities include the large, hyperchromic nuclei with occasional mitotic figures.

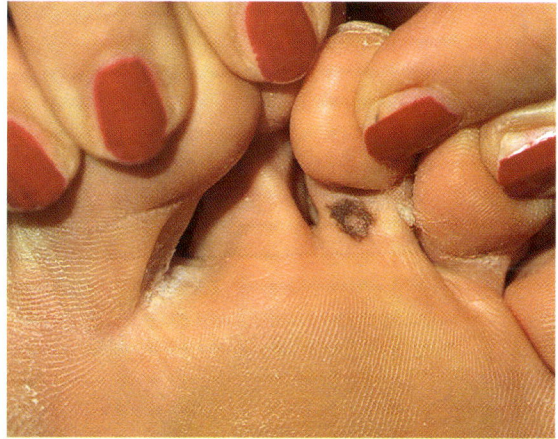

(b)

Differential diagnosis

Malignant melanoma must be differentiated histologically.

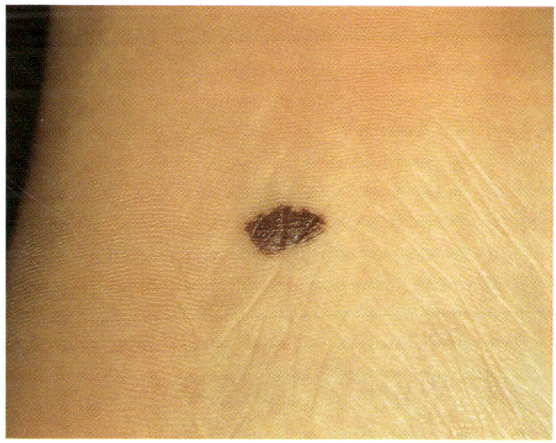

Figure 2.46(a–c)
Dysplastic naevi. Dysplastic naevi are asymmetrical, poorly-defined lesions of more than 6 mm in diameter that vary in colour from different shades of brown to black.

(c)

Clinical features: Spitz naevi

Clinical

On the feet, Spitz naevi present as solitary lesions that vary greatly in colour (from pink to black). The surface configuration of the naevi can either be flat topped or papillomatous when occurring on the dorsal aspects of the foot. Spitz naevi most often affect children and young adults but may appear at almost any stage of life. In children these naevi are usually smooth, firm, asymptomatic nodules, which are pink or red in colour because they are highly vascular. The lesion may grow rapidly and may attain a diameter of 1–2 cm. In older patients Spitz naevi may assume a brown, dark-brown or uniform black colour.

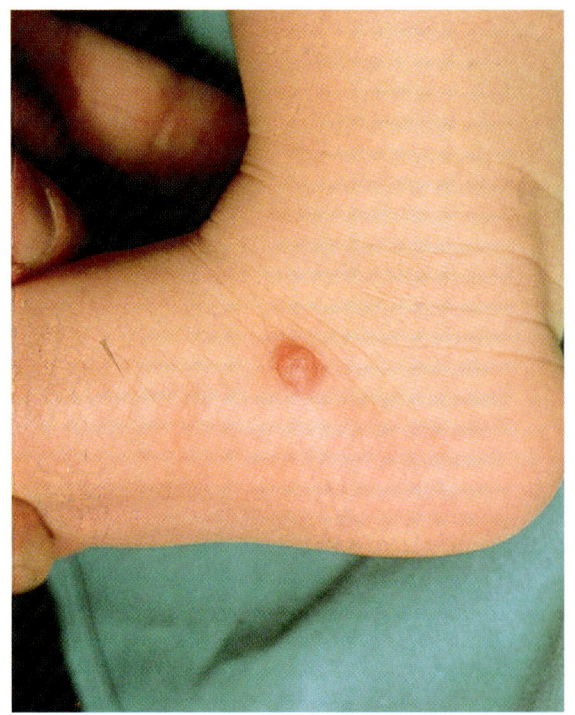

(a)

Histopathological

Spitz naevi are characterized by melanocytes with large nuclei and round, oval, polygonal or spindle-shaped. Multinucleated or mononuclear giant melanocytes, are commonly seen. The melanocytes may have atypical nuclei and may demonstrate mitotic figures. The overlying epidermis may be thickened, and homogeneous, pink globules (Kamino bodies) may be observed at the dermo-epidermal junction.

Differential diagnosis

Hemangiomas are not as firm and blanch on diascopy.

Solitary mastocytomas are marked by a yellow or orange line and burn when rubbed.

Juvenile xanthogranulomas are hard, and yellow in colour.

Malignant melanomas (pigmented lesions after puberty) require histopathology for differentiation.

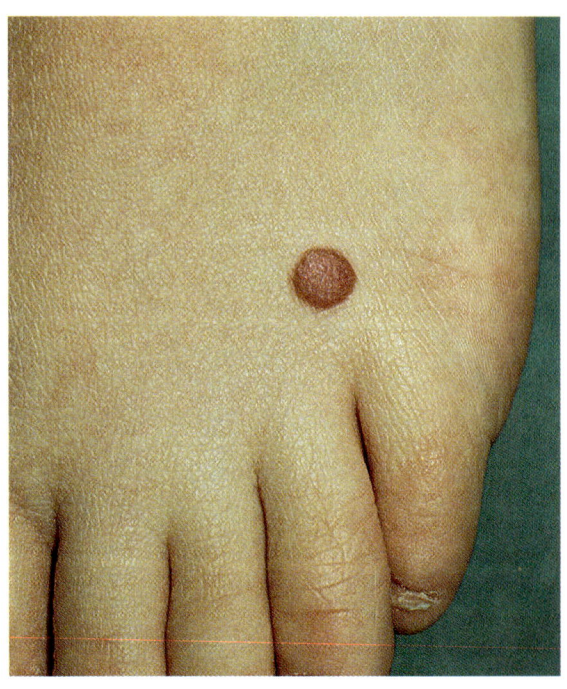

(b)

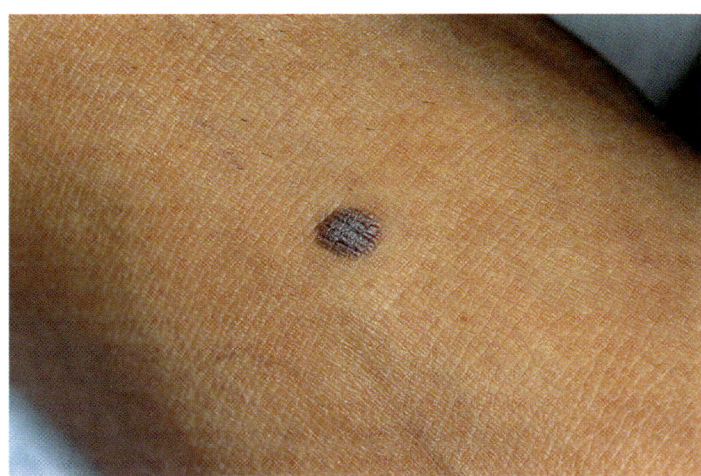

(c)

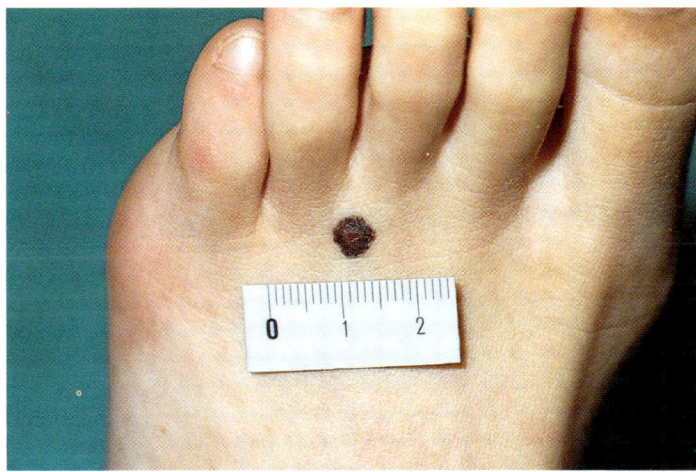

(d)

Figure 2.47(a–d)

Spitz naevi. Spitz naevi appear as solitary, smooth, firm, asymptomatic nodules that may grow rapidly to attain a diameter of 1–2 cm. In young patients the lesions are pink (a) or reddish brown (b), while in older patients they may be dark brown (c) or black (d).

Clinical features: Blue naevi

Clinical

Blue naevi consist of well demarcated, smooth, usually slightly–raised, solitary macules or papules (common blue naevi) or nodules (cellular blue naevi) that vary in colour from a bluish-grey to blue-black. The dorsal aspect of the foot is one of the sites of predilection. The majority of these lesions appear in the second decade of life.

Histopathological

Accumulations of pigmented, spindle-shaped melanocytes will be observed in the dermis and/or subcutaneous fat.

Differential diagnosis

Blue rubber-bleb naevi are nipple-shaped, and are tender, rubbery and compressible to the touch.

Solitary glomus tumours are extremely rare.

In malignant melanoma a blue-black pigmentation is usually mixed in with various shades of reddish-brown.

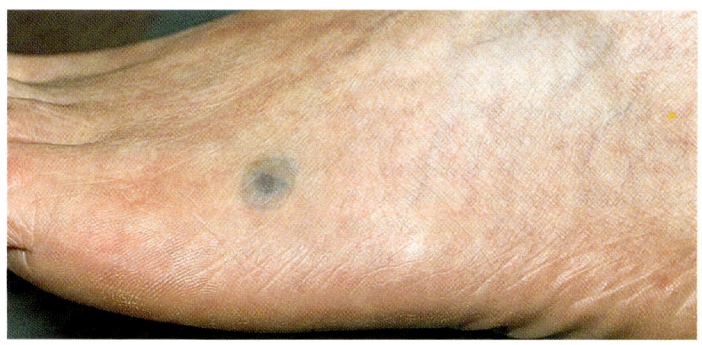

(a)

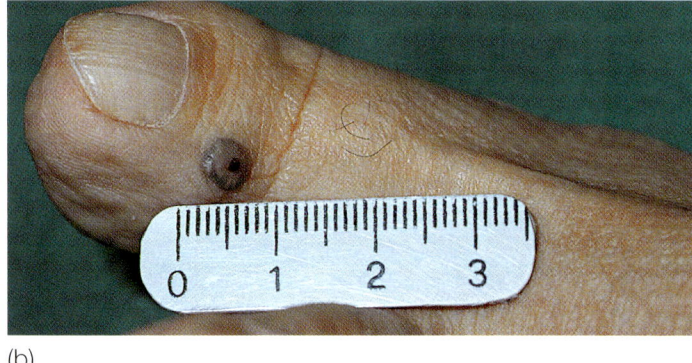

(b)

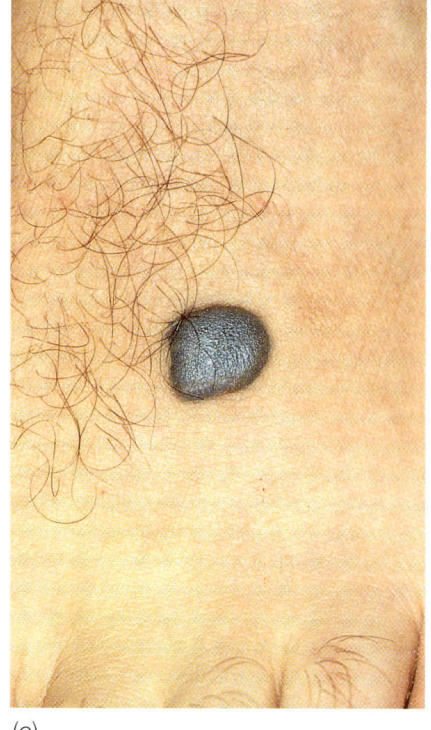

(c)

Figure 2.48(a–c)

Blue naevi. Blue naevi are smooth, well demarcated papules or nodules that vary in colour from bluish-grey (a and b) to blue-black (c). The dorsal aspect of the feet is one of the sites of predilection.

PEUTZ–JEGHERS SYNDROME

Peutz–Jeghers syndrome (or periorificial lentiginosis) is an autosomal dominant disorder characterized by mucocutaneous pigmentation and hamartomatous polyps in the gastrointestinal tract. The pigmented lesions may develop at birth or in early childhood and are located in the buccal mucosa, on the lips and in the perioral region. The hands and feet may be affected. Histologically the lesions consist of increased numbers of dendritic melanocytes arranged as solitary units at the dermo-epidermal junction of a hyperpigmented epidermis.

Clinical features

The lesions are usually found on the soles and appear as dark brown or black macules that are round or oval in shape.

Differential diagnosis

Plantar naevi may easily be ruled out because of the absence of pigmentary lesions in the oral mucosa and of gastrointestinal polyps.

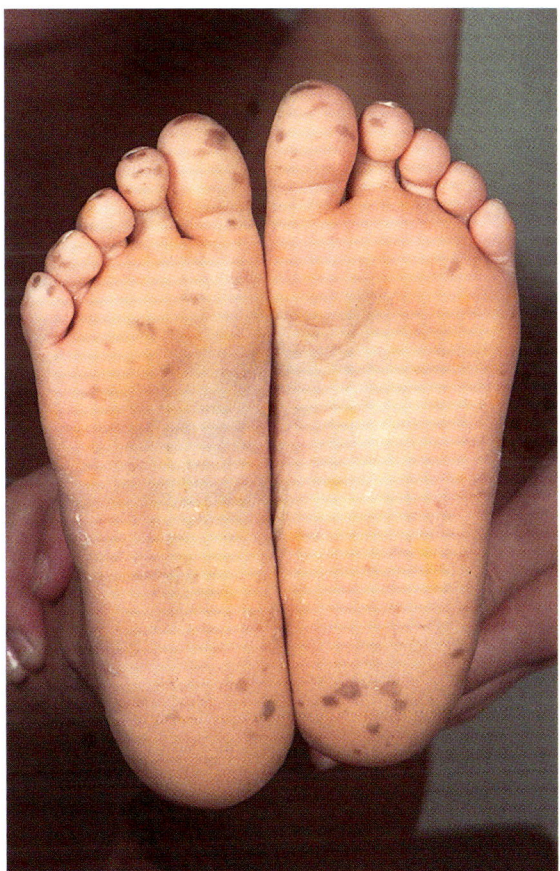

Figure 2.49

Peutz–Jeghers syndrome. This condition presents with dark brown macules irregularly distributed on the soles.

MALIGNANT MELANOMA

Malignant melanoma (MM) is a malignant tumour that arises from melanocytes. MM usually begins as a proliferation of atypical epidermal melanocytes that may extend into the dermis and subcutaneous tissue. Clinical features helpful in identifying a MM and common to all variants of MM are:

- pigmented lesions that grow insidiously, either rapidly or slowly, and that change in size and shape (asymmetry of the lesions, irregular borders, a diameter of 7 mm, nodular growth);
- a change in colour: defined by a variegated colour that can be either pink, red, brown, black, blue or white;
- inflammation, ulceration, bleeding and itching.

These features may be summarized by the ABCD mnemonic: A (asymmetry), B (borders), C (colour), D (diameter).

The four main clinical subdivisions of MM are subungual malignant melanoma, superficial spreading melanoma, nodular melanoma and acral lentiginous melanoma.

The main histopathological findings of MM at all anatomic sites are asymmetry, poor circumscription, failure of maturation of melanocytes with progressive descent into the dermis and single-cell invasion or prominent pagetoid nests within the epidermis. Cytologic features of importance are nuclear abnormalities and an increased number of mitotic figures. A lymphocytic inflammatory response may be seen in the underlying dermis.

Clinical features: acral lentiginous melanoma (ALM)

ALM involves, by definition, the palms of the hands and the soles of the feet, with the sole being the most commonly infected site. ALM represents approximately 50% of all melanomas of the foot. This type of melanoma is relatively infrequent among Caucasians (10%) but represents 50% of all melanomas among blacks and Asians.

ALM mainly affects older patients (median age 65 years) and is characterized by a pigmented macular lesion, 1–3 cm or more in diameter with irregular borders and of various colours. A bluish colour indicates a dense melanin pigmentation in the dermis. Amelanotic lesions usually appear red in colour. In time, raised black nodules may develop within this macular area of pigmentation. Also, if these lesions are slightly raised they may be deeply invasive. Pruritus, pain and bleeding may be symptoms associated with these lesions. Plantar melanomas occur most frequently on the weight-bearing areas, particularly on the heel (45%).

Differential diagnosis

Acral lentiginous naevi (dysplastic naevi) must be differentiated histologically.

Compound naevi are round or oval, sharply demarcated, homogeneously pigmented and 3–6 mm in diameter.

Plantar warts with thrombosed capillaries, black heel ('talon-noir') (haemorrhages following trauma) and vascular lesions are easily ruled out by epiluminescence.

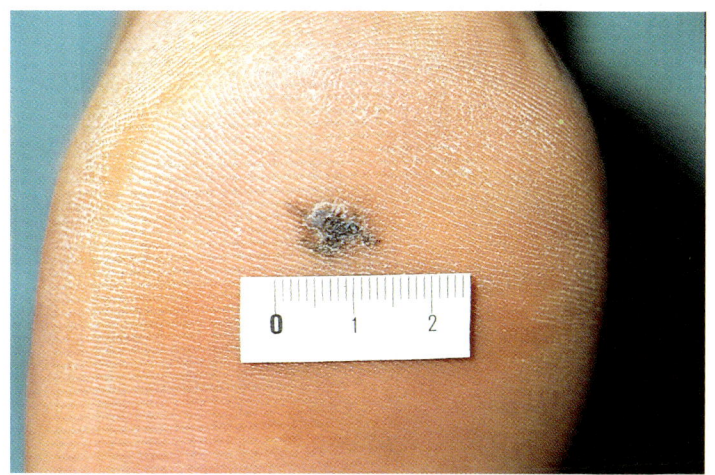
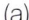

(a)

Figure 2.50(a–c)
Acral lentiginous melanoma. These plantar melanomas present here as irregular, black lesions 1–3 cm in length.

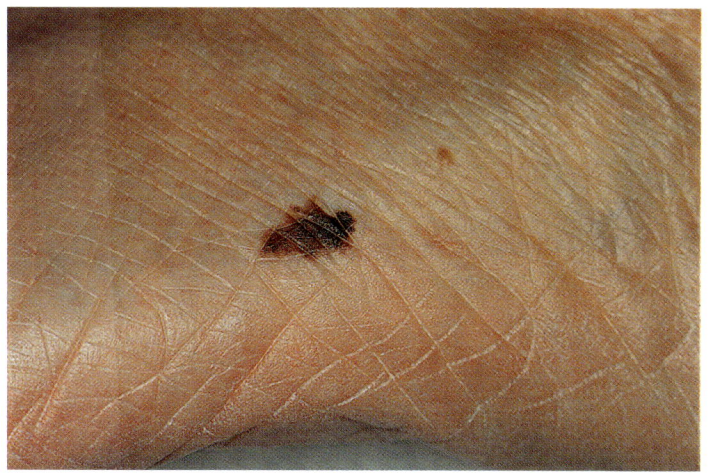

(b)

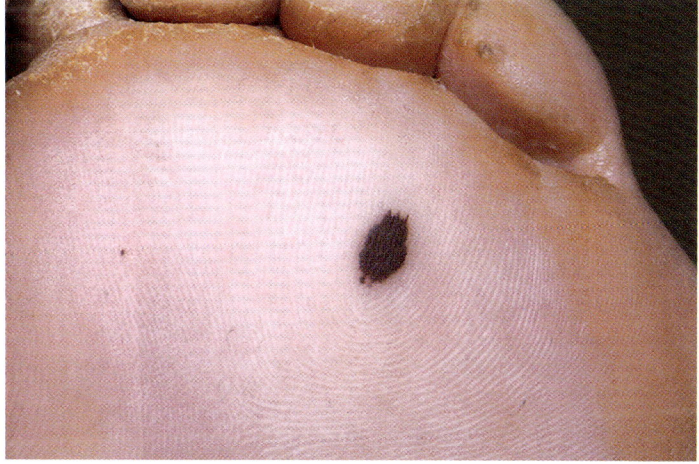

(c)

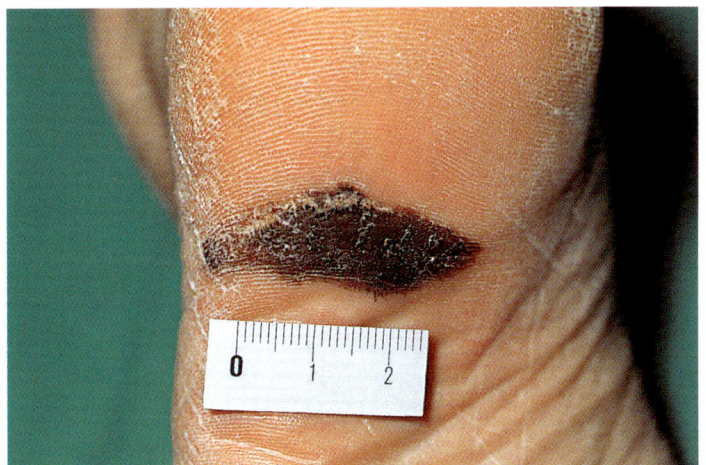

Figure 2.51(a–c)

Acral lentiginous melanoma. These large, plantar melanomas demonstrate the irregular shapes and, in two of them (b and c), varying colours typical of this disease.

(a)

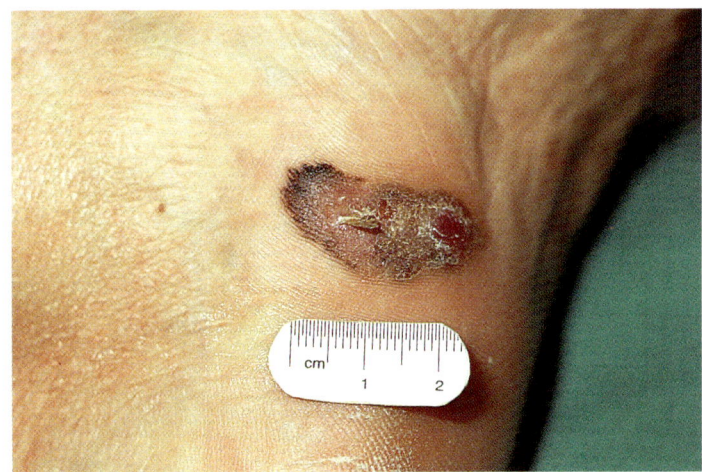

(b)

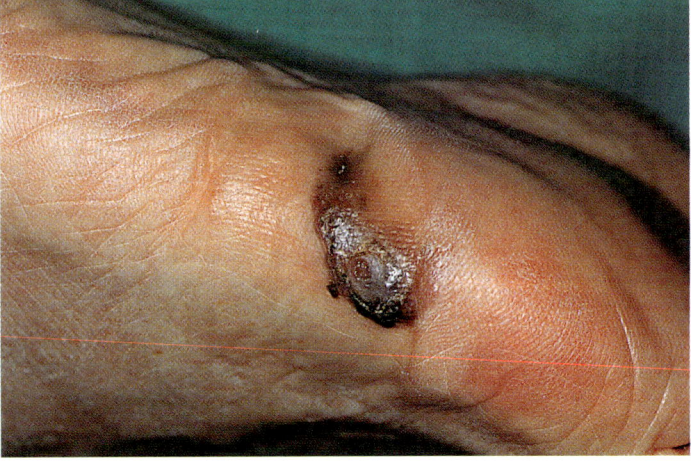

(c)

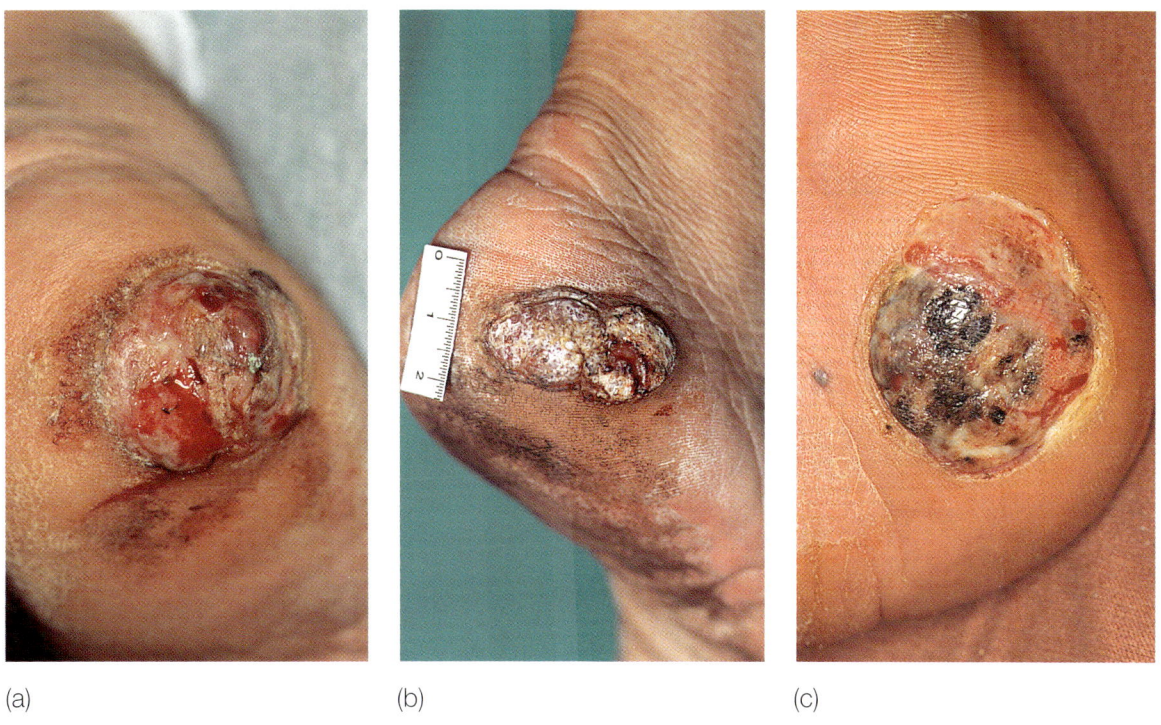

(a)   (b)   (c)

Figure 2.52(a–c)

Acral lentiginous melanoma. Plantar melanomas occur most frequently on weight-bearing areas, particularly the heel.

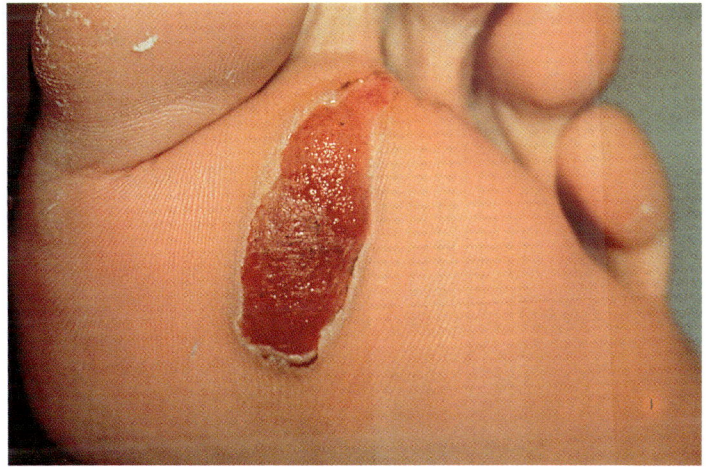

Figure 2.53

Acral lentiginous melanoma. Plantar amelanotic melanomas are usually red in colour.

Clinical features: Subungual malignant melanoma

Subungual or periungual malignant melanoma may be regarded as a variant of ALM. It may present as an irregular discolouration of the nail-bed and nail-plate, with splitting and progressive destruction of the nail. The presence of pigment on the nail-fold distal to the nail (Hutchinson's sign) as a result of leaching of pigment into the paronychial area is strongly suggestive of subungual malignant melanoma. The first toe is the area most commonly affected.

Differential diagnosis

Fungal infections with nail pigmentations are easily differentiated by the absence of Hutchinson's sign and by positive microscopic examination and culture.

Subungual haematoma has a history of trauma; there is also usually a lack of pigment on the nail-fold.

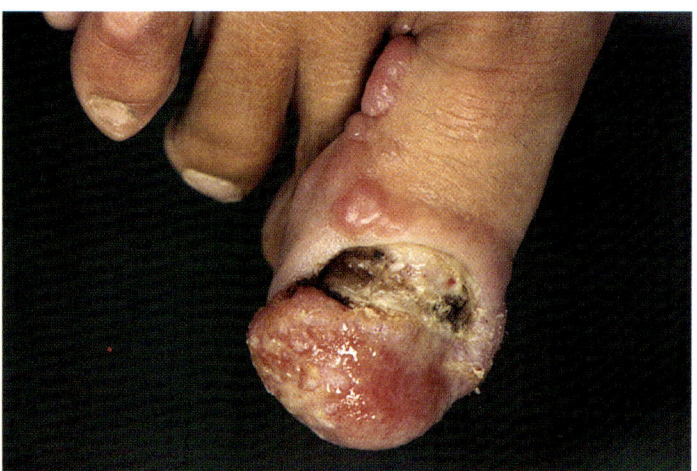

(a)

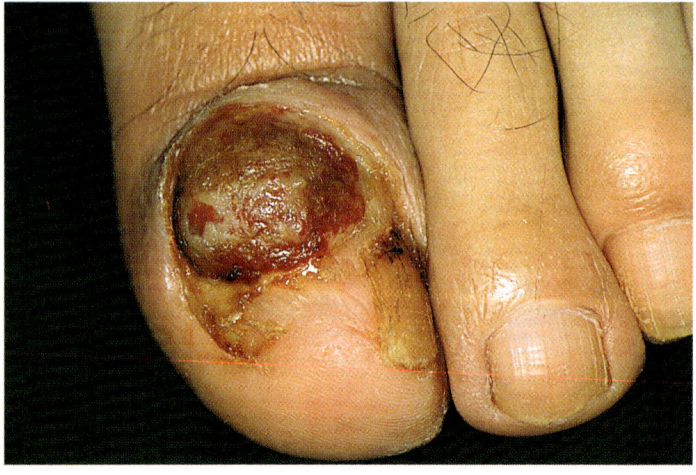

(b)

Figure 2.54(a,b)
Subungual malignant melanoma.
An advanced subungual melanoma has caused destruction of the nail. The nail-fold is pigmented (Hutchinson's sign). The big toe is the usual site of invasion. (Photograph courtesy of Professor Aldo Finzi.)

Clinical features: Superficial spreading melanoma

Superficial spreading melanoma (SSM) may occur on both the dorsal and plantar aspects of the feet. It appears first as flat, pigmented lesions that grow gradually to display irregular borders, variegation in colour and skin infiltration. The lesions' colour might contain combinations of pink, brown, red, white, blue and black lines. Nodules may develop within a SSM which indicates vertical growth.

Differential diagnosis

Acquired and congenital melanocytic naevi are symmetrical, usually less than 10 mm in diameter and have regular borders. Although most melanocytic lesions have various shades of brown, red, blue-black or white, the appearance of lines is suggestive of an SSM. Because diagnosis sometimes cannot be made clinically or by epiluminescence, histopathology is necessary.

Pigmented basal-cell carcinomas present with characteristic rolled, translucent borders and telangiectases, and their colour is uniform.

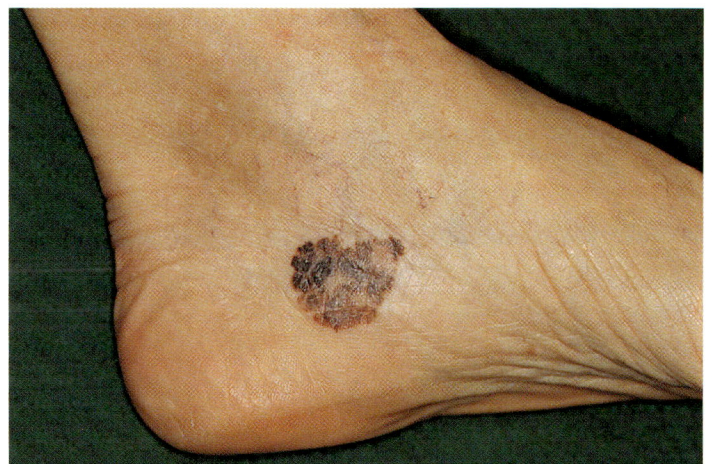

(a)

Figure 2.55(a,b)

Superficial spreading melanoma. This presents as flat, irregularly-shaped, pigmented lesions that vary in colour (pink, brown, white, red, blue or black). The development of nodules within an SSM (b) is suggestive of vertical growth.

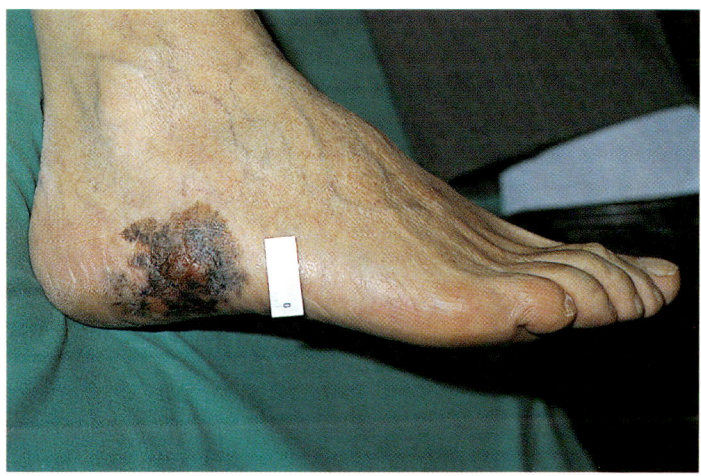

(b)

Clinical features: Nodular melanoma

Nodular melanoma (NM) rarely occurs on the feet and is only occasionally observed on the soles. NM manifests as a raised, dome-shaped, reddish-brown to blue-black nodule. This lesion grows rapidly and is frequently associated with ulceration and bleeding. NM may lack melanin (amelanotic NM) and may be red in colour.

Differential diagnosis

Vascular tumours (pyogenic granuloma, thrombosed haemangioma) are ruled out by epiluminescence and, if necessary, by histopathology.

Blue naevi are clinically stable lesions: they do not vary in colour or size.

Eccrine poroma is usually seen on the soles and presents as a moist, pink nodule. Diagnostic histopathology is recommended.

Histiocytoma is firm, and yellowish-brown in colour.

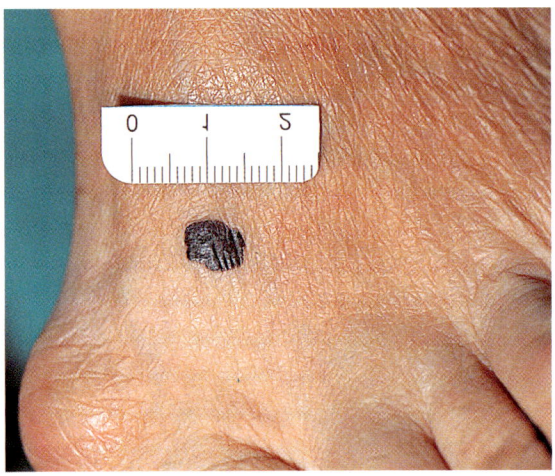

(a)

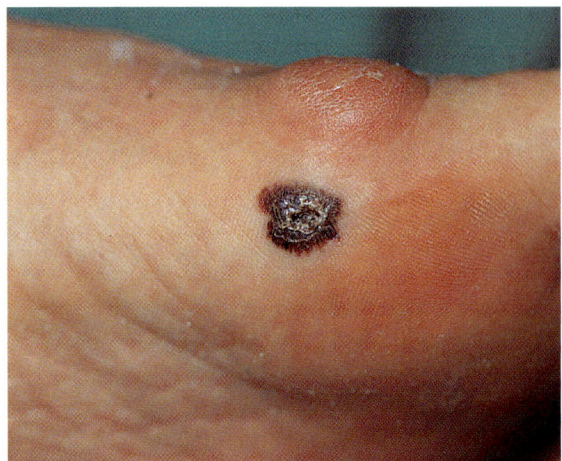

(b)

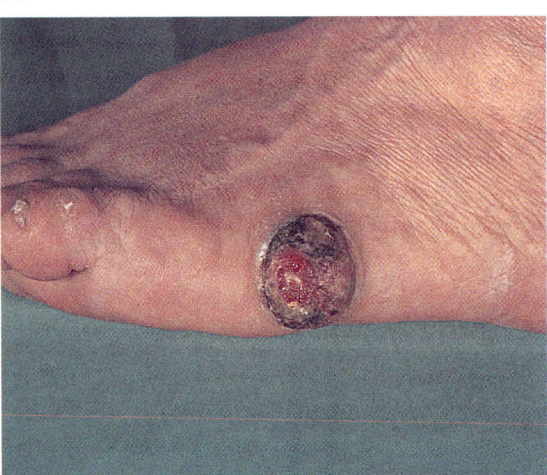

(c)

Figure 2.56(a–c)

Nodular melanoma. Nodular melanomas occur as raised, dome-shaped, reddish-brown to black nodules. These may ulcerate (c). Such lesions rarely occur on the feet.

LANGERHANS' CELL HISTIOCYTOSIS

Langerhans' cell histiocytosis (LCH) is a disease of unknown aetiology characterized by the proliferation of a distinct cell type (S100+ and CD1a+) whose cytoplasm contains Langerhans' granules. LCH has four main clinical forms: Letterer–Siwe disease, Hand–Schüler–Christian disease, eosinophilic granuloma and Hashimoto–Pritzker disease.

Lesions on the feet have occasionally been seen only in Letterer–Siwe disease and in Hashimoto–Pritzker disease.

Clinical features

Letterer–Siwe disease (LSD) is the acute, disseminated form of LCH characterized by papular scaly lesions on the trunk and scalp. These lesions may become vesicular, pustular and even purpuric. Infection of the soles is very rare, consisting of scattered, purpuric papules and papular pustules. The appearance of petechiae at this site is a poor sign for prognosis.

Hashimoto–Pritzker disease (HPD) is the benign, self-healing form of LCH characterized by the presence at birth of multiple, disseminated, elevated, firm, reddish-brown nodules that rapidly resolve spontaneously.

Differential diagnosis

The papulopustular lesions of LSD must be differentiated from scabies (presence of mites and eggs when scraped) infantile acropustulosis (presence of pruritus and eosinophilia; histologic examination is necessary), candidiasis (presence of hyphae or pseudohyphae), pustular psoriasis (very rare in early infancy; crops of pustules within areas of erythema) and hand-foot-and-mouth disease (oblong vesicles, involvement of oral mucosa).

The nodular lesions of HPD need differentiation from juvenile xanthogranuloma (yellow in colour; spontaneous resolution in several years), pyogenic granuloma (bleeds easily; surrounded by a collar of acanthotic epidermis), Spitz naevus (usually solitary, pink to red in colour; histopathology may be necessary), diffuse neonatal haemangiomatosis (cherry-like soft lesions; histopathology is necessary) and mastocytosis (whealing after rubbing).

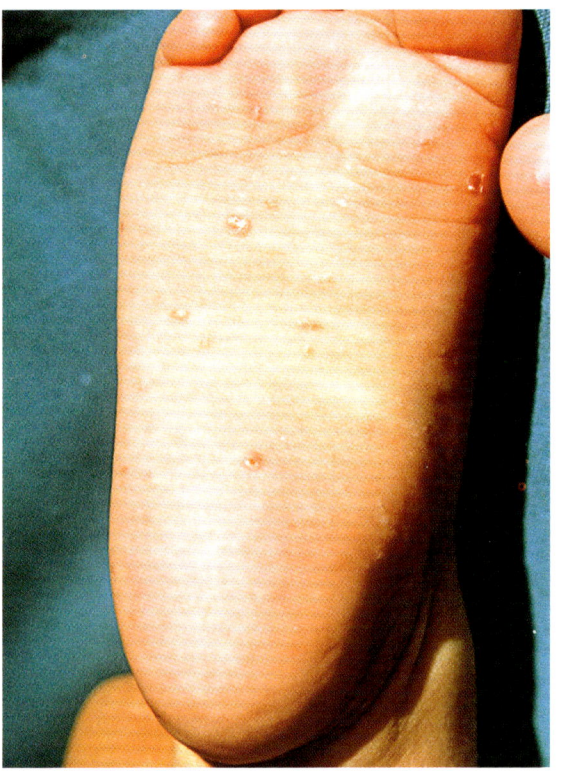

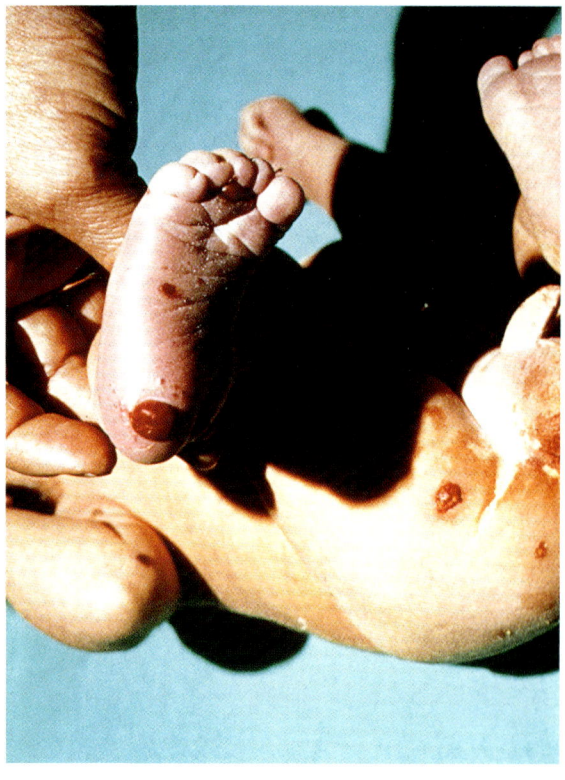

Figure 2.57

Langerhans' cell histiocytosis: Letterer–Siwe disease. Papules and papular pustules are present on the sole of this infant. Involvement of the feet is very rare.

Figure 2.58

Langerhans' cell histiocytosis: Hashimoto–Pritzker disease. These firm, reddish-brown, elevated nodules were present at birth and disappeared spontaneously within 6 months.

JUVENILE XANTHOGRANULOMA

Juvenile xanthogranuloma (JXG) is a benign, self-healing, non-Langerhans' cell histiocytosis most frequently seen in infants and children. Two main clinical variants can be distinguished: a small nodular form and a large nodular form. Involvement of the feet has only been described in the micronodular form.

Clinical features

The condition manifests as hemispheric, firm lesions, 2–5 mm in diameter that are reddish-brown at first, but that rapidly acquire a yellow line. Localization on the plantar aspect of the feet is extremely rare.

Differential diagnosis

Mastocytosis (urticaria pigmentosa) may be distinguished by the absence of the yellow shadow and the presence of Darier's sign.

Spitz naevus may be reddish-brown or orange but never yellow. Histopathology may be necessary.

Tuberous xanthomas appear only in hyperlipidemic states.

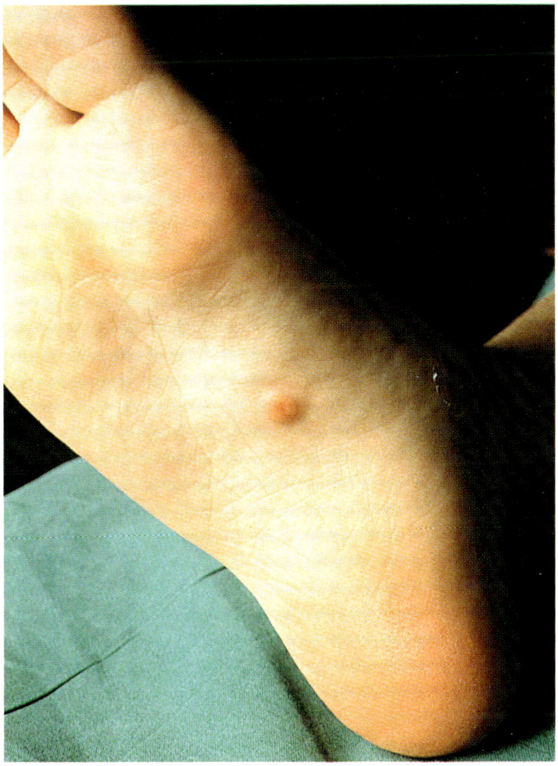

Figure 2.59

Juvenile xanthogranuloma. Hemispheric, yellowish-brown, firm nodules can be observed on the sole. They rarely appear on plantar aspect of the feet.

MASTOCYTOSIS

The term 'mastocytosis' refers to a spectrum of disorders characterized by the proliferation of mast cells. The main clinical forms of cutaneous mastocytosis are: solitary mastocytoma, disseminated mastocytosis (or urticaria pigmentosa) and diffuse mastocytosis. These are, in the main, paediatric, benign, self-healing conditions. The feet may be involved in all the variants. Typical of this disease is Darier's sign – the whealing of the lesions after rubbing.

Disseminated mastocytosis (urticaria pigmentosa) needs differentiation from urticaria (brown colour lacking; lesions move from site to site), nodular scabies (refer to the patient's personal and family history) and the micronodular form of JXG (yellow in colour; absence of Darier's sign).

Incontinentia pigmenti and epidermolysis bullosa can mimic the diffuse form of mastocytosis. In incontinentia pigmenti, blisters follow Blaschko's lines and are replaced rapidly by verrucous lesions. In epidermolysis bullosa, the skin is not infiltrated by mast cells.

Clinical features

Solitary mastocytoma is usually present at birth as a round or oval nodule up to 3–4 cm in diameter. Its colour varies from that of the surrounding skin to yellow or brown and its surface usually resembles the pitted skin of an orange. Serous or haemorrhagic bullae are formed readily. The soles are always spared.

In disseminated mastocytosis (urticaria pigmentosa) maculopapular lesions may occasionally be observed on the soles.

Diffuse mastocytosis occurs almost exclusively in infants and is characterized by the diffuse infiltration of the entire skin. The skin appears thickened, is marked by deep furrows and is a reddish-brown colour. Blisters occur frequently and itching is severe.

Differential diagnosis

Solitary mastocytoma must be differentiated from the macronodular form of JXG (yellow in colour; absence of Darier's sign), Hashimoto–Pritzker disease (absence of Darier's sign; histopathological examination necessary) and pseudolymphomas (e.g. insect bites; histopathological examination necessary).

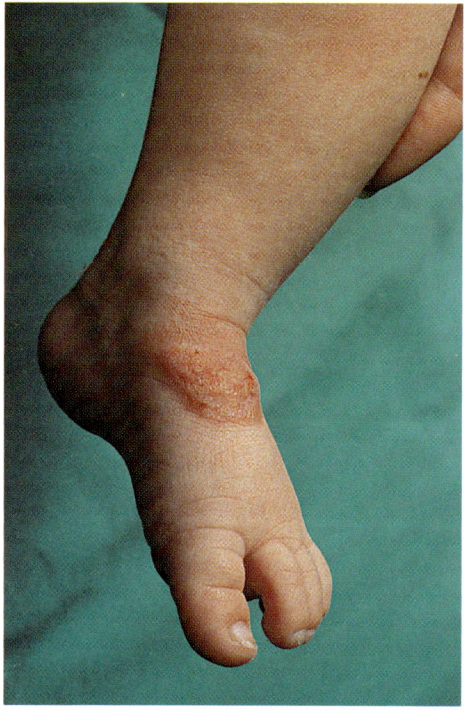

Figure 2.60

Solitary mastocytosis. This solitary plaque is reddish-brown in colour, is relatively well demarcated and its surface resembles the pitted skin of an orange. Urtication after the lesion has been rubbed is known as Darier's sign.

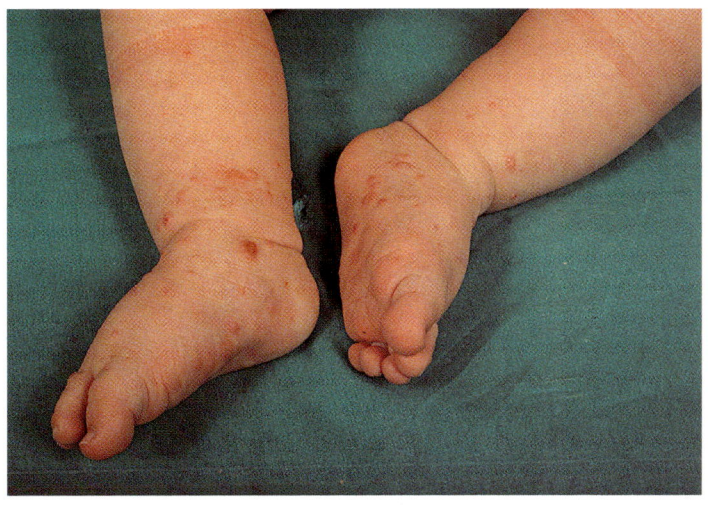

(a)

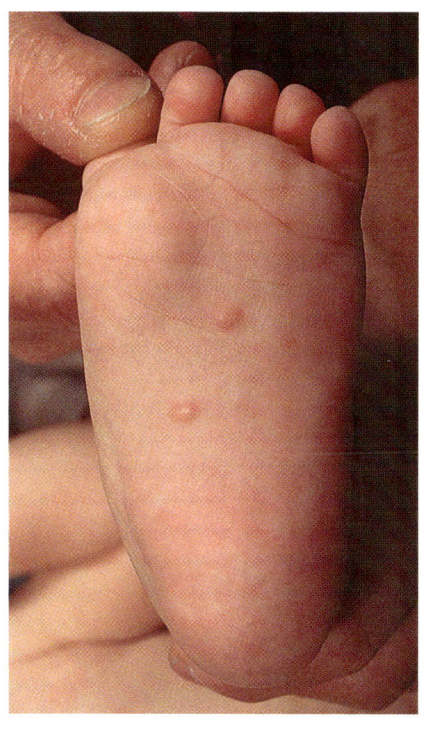

(b)

Figure 2.61(a,b)

Disseminated mastocytosis (urticaria pigmentosa). In this mastocytosis, micronodular, reddish-brown lesions are distributed irregularly on the feet.

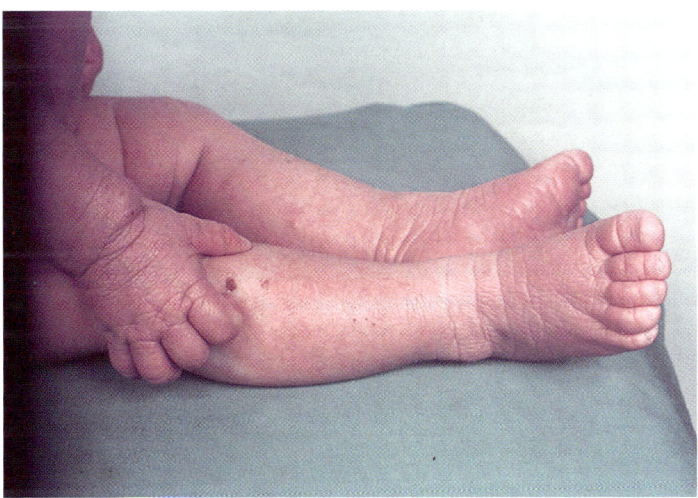

Figure 2.62

Diffuse mastocytosis (pachyerythrodermic form). The skin is diffusely infiltrated and appears thickened. It is marked by deep furrows.

SARCOMAS

Epithelioid sarcoma

Epithelioid sarcoma is a rare malignant tumour of the connective tissue that favours the acral regions of young adults. It appears as skin-coloured to reddish-brown, firm-subcutaneous, non-tender nodules. Ulcerations or sinus formations may be present. The course of the disease is usually unrelentless, leading to death from metastasis. Histologically it consists of epithelioid cells with abundant, deeply eosinophilic, often vacuolated cytoplasm around foci of necrosis. Mitotic figures are common.

Fibrosarcoma

Fibrosarcoma is an uncommon tumour of the connective tissue that is composed of spindle cells resembling fibroblasts. The tumour can occur anywhere and presents as a smooth, firm, reddish-brown nodule that becomes more vascular and purpuric as it grows. Necrosis and ulcerations occur frequently. Fibrosarcomas readily metastasize through lymphatic and blood vessels. Histologically, the tumour is composed of anaplastic spindle cells that are often polymorphic and that frequently have mitotic figures arranged randomly.

Malignant fibrous histiocytoma

Malignant fibrous histiocytoma is a polymorphic sarcoma that has the ability to produce collagen in the form of a large, irregular nodule or plaque in the underlying dermis. The majority of malignant fibrous histiocytomas that have been reported to date have been located on the extremities of patients aged 50 years or older. Previous radiotherapies or burn scars seem to predispose to these tumours. About one-third of the tumours metastasize within 2 years. Histologically the tumour consists of spindle cells and irregularly-shaped cells, with many mitoses arranged in different patterns: storiform, myxoid, inflammatory, giant cell and angiomatoid.

Angiosarcoma

Angiosarcoma is a malignant vascular tumour that arises from both the vascular and lymphatic endothelium. In the latter case, angiosarcomas are associated with congenital lymphoedema of the lower limbs or lymphoedema secondary to a filarial infection. The lesions are characterized by areas of lividity or violaceous nodules that increase in number and size rapidly and that may ulcerate. In the majority of cases, these tumours are fatal. Histologically, the well differentiated tumours appear as irregular vascular spaces that form an intricate network of freely anastomosing vessels. These vessels contain erythrocytes with extensive fragmentation of collagen. Atypical endothelial cells may become syncytial.

Differential diagnosis

Many proliferative and inflammatory disorders must be taken into consideration in differential diagnosis (fibromatoses, sarcoidosis, subcutaneous granuloma annulare, sporotrichosis, nocardiasis, etc). Histopathology is necessary.

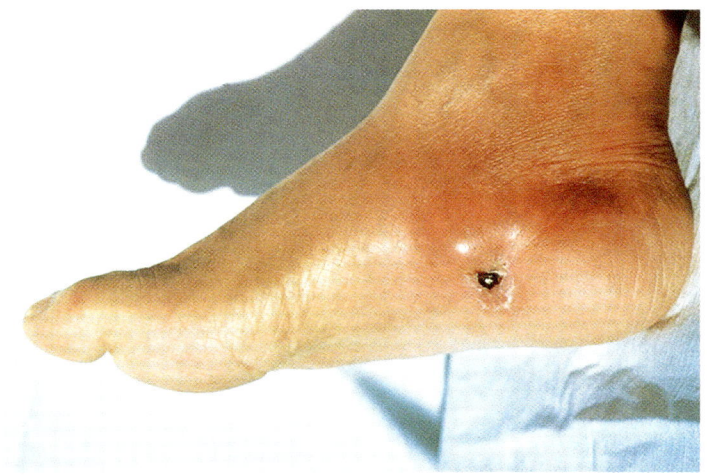

Figure 2.63

Epithelioid sarcoma. This sarcoma presents as a reddish-brown, firm, subcutaneous plaque with a small central ulceration that is covered by a crust.

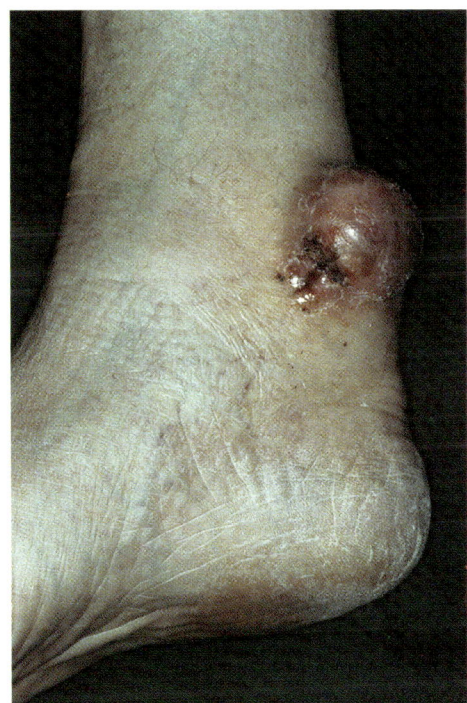

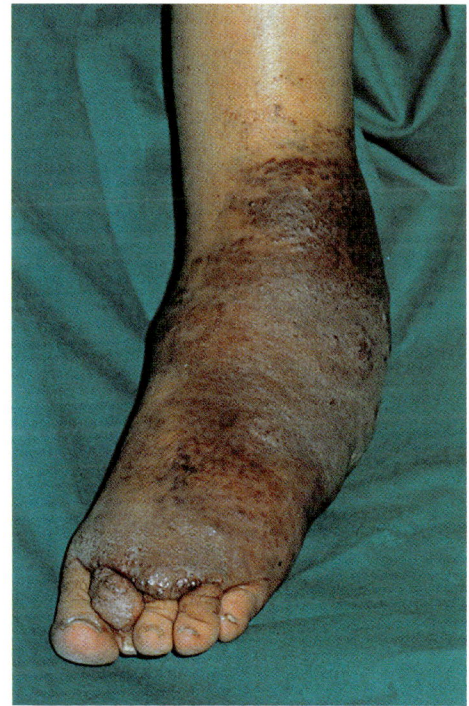

Figure 2.64

Malignant fibrous histiocytoma. This histiocytoma is a large, irregular, firm, reddish-violet nodule that is partially ulcerated. (Photograph courtesy of Professor Aldo Finzi.)

Figure 2.65

Angiosarcoma. This angiomatous plaque on the dorsal aspect of a foot is the result of the merging of reddish violaceous nodules that rapidly increased in size and number.

MYCOSIS FUNGOIDES

Mycosis fungoides (MF) is a primarily cutaneous T-cell lymphoma that occurs as a result of proliferation of helper T-cells. Skin lesions consist of round, oval or arciform, more or less infiltrated plaques, and nodules and tumours with or without randomly distributed ulcers. In cases of diffuse involvement, the skin may become erythrodermic. Histologically the disease is characterized by a diffuse, band-like lymphocytic infiltrate in the upper dermis. The cells are extremely polymorphic. Pautrier's microabscesses are also found in the epidermis – they are small groups of mononuclear cells surrounded by a halo-like clear space.

Clinical features

In 11.5% of patients, the feet may be involved at some stage during the course of the disease (mainly in the erythrodermic form). In these cases the skin is diffusely red, infiltrated and scaling.

Mycosis fungoides palmaris et plantaris in an uncommon form of the disease that primarily manifests itself on the palms and on the soles. Clinically it may mimic various inflammatory dermatoses.

On the soles, skin lesions may be diffuse, vesiculopustular or hyperkeratotic, or may present as solitary nodules or warty plaques.

Differential diagnosis

MF on the feet may mimic many dermatoses, such as contact dermatitis, psoriasis, pityriasis rubra pilaris, dermatophyte infection, warts and hypertrophic lichen planus. These diseases may be ruled out by the histopathological, immunohistochemical and molecular findings typical of MF.

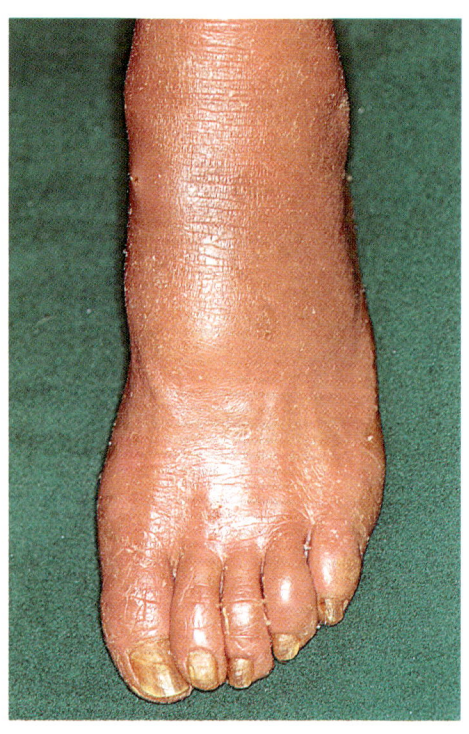

(a)

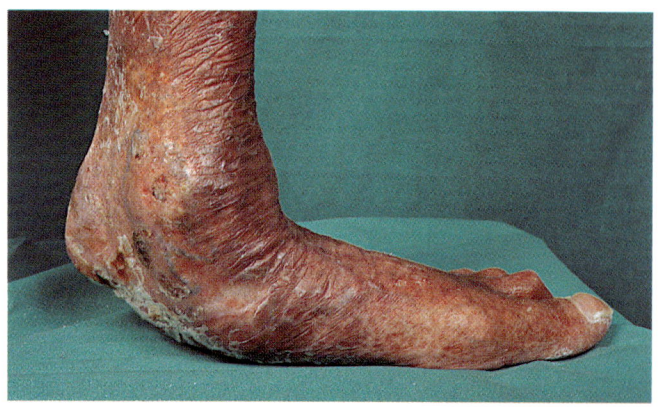

(b)

Figure 2.66(a,b)

Mycosis fungoides. On the feet mycosis fungoides may present as infiltrated plaques (a), or in its erythrodermic form, as a diffuse, red, scaling infiltration (b). (Photograph courtesy of Professor Aldo Finzi.)

METASTASIS OF THE TOES

Phalangeal metastases are a very rare occurrence, perhaps because of the absence of red bone marrow in the acral bones. Metastases most commonly affect the distal phalange of the first toe, which appears swollen, tender and erythematous but is not painful. Less commonly, reddish purple, dome-shaped, verrucous or ulcerated nodules may occur. Most metastatic lesions seem initially to involve bone and, subsequently, the soft tissues, while adjacent joints are spared. Phalangeal metastases have been mainly reported in men with a mean age of 55 years. Tumours of the genitourinary tract seem to be the most common source of foot metastases. In these patients prognosis is generally very poor (only a few months).

Differential diagnosis

Metastatic lesions in the digits must be differentiated from infections, gout, rheumatoid arthritis, primary tumours of the nail unit, malignant melanoma, leukaemia and plasma cell myeloma.

The discrepancy between clinical signs and the degree of pain, the lack of response to specific treatments or to surgical drainage, and radiological findings (well-defined osteolytic lesions without the involvement of the joint cartilage and the joint space) should confirm the suspicion of metastatic malignancies.

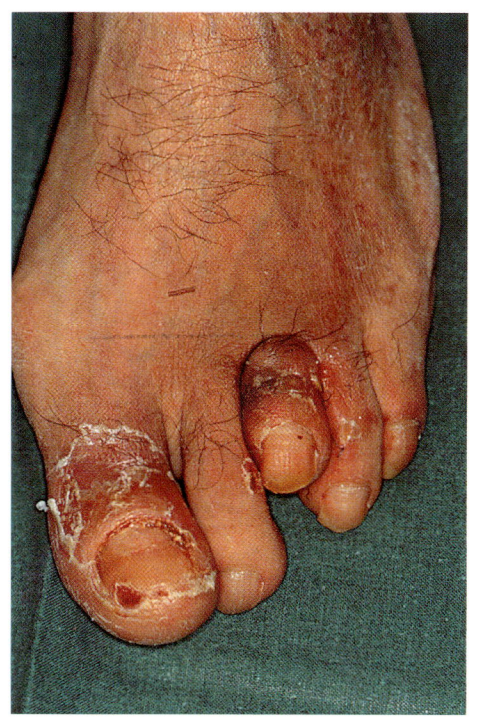

Figure 2.67

Metastasis of the toes. In this patient with a malignant tumour, two phalangeal metastases occurred on the first and third toes as erythematous and tender, but not painful, nodules. (Photograph courtesy of Professor Antonella Tosti.)

3 Hereditary and keratinization disorders

PALMOPLANTAR HEREDITARY KERATODERMAS
VERRUCOUS EPIDERMAL NAEVI
INFLAMMATORY LINEAR VERRUCOUS NAEVUS
POROKERATOSIS
PITYRIASIS RUBRA PILARIS
DARIER'S DISEASE
EPIDERMODYSPLASIA VERRUCIFORMIS
HEREDITARY EPIDERMOLYSIS BULLOSA
INCONTINENTIA PIGMENTI
ACRODERMATITIS ENTEROPATHICA

PALMOPLANTAR HEREDITARY KERATODERMAS

Palmoplantar hereditary keratodermas (PPHK) are a heterogeneous group of genodermatoses that can be divided into two forms: diffuse and focal.

Diffuse PPHK

PPHK Thost–Unna

This is thought to be the most common PPHK. It usually manifests at 2–5 years of age with a diffuse erythema. Hyperkeratosis then commences at the margins of the soles and extends to the centre. The disease is bilateral, symmetrical and has no tendency to spread to extensor surfaces. Initially, it has sharp borders surrounded by an erythematous halo. Marked hyperhidrosis is usual. Histologically, the disorder is characterized by compact hyperkeratosis, hypergranulosis and moderate acanthosis. It is determined by an autosomal dominant gene.

Epidermolytic PPHK Vörner

This keratoderma resembles Thost–Unna clinically but hyperhidrosis is not a common finding. The disease is inherited via an autosomal dominant trait.

Progressive PPHK Greither

This autosomal dominant disorder is characterized by diffuse keratoderma with hyperhidrosis extending to the dorsal aspect of the feet (transgrediens pattern). In addition, keratotic patches may develop on the limbs (progrediens pattern). The disease tends to improve spontaneously in middle age. It differs essentially from Mal de Meleda by its dominant mode of inheritance.

Mal de Meleda

A very rare transgrediens, this is a progressive form of PPHK comprising a 'glove and sock' hyperkeratosis that does not usually have sharply-defined margins. Hyperkeratotic plaques may occasionally appear, especially on the elbows and knees. Hyperhidrosis with maceration and maleoder is always present. This disease is very similar to progressive PPHK Greither but is persistent and is inherited as a recessive trait. Histopathologically, Mal de Meleda is characterized by epidermal hyperplasia, hyperkeratosis and inflammatory infiltrate around the dermal vessels.

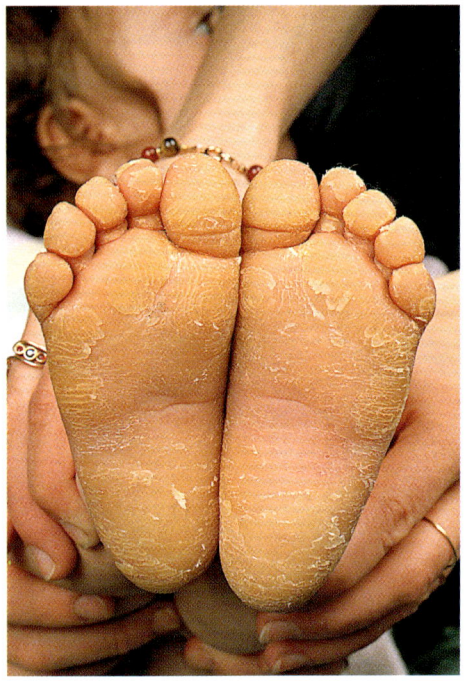

(a)

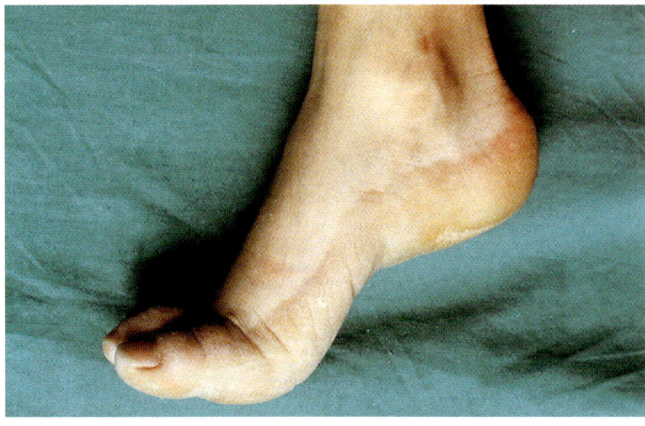

(b)

Figure 3.1(a,b)

Diffuse palmoplantar hereditary keratoderma (PPHK): Thost–Unna disease. Diffuse involvement of the soles is apparent by the yellowish hyperkeratosis (a). Note the sharp demarcation of the keratoderma on the side of the foot (b).

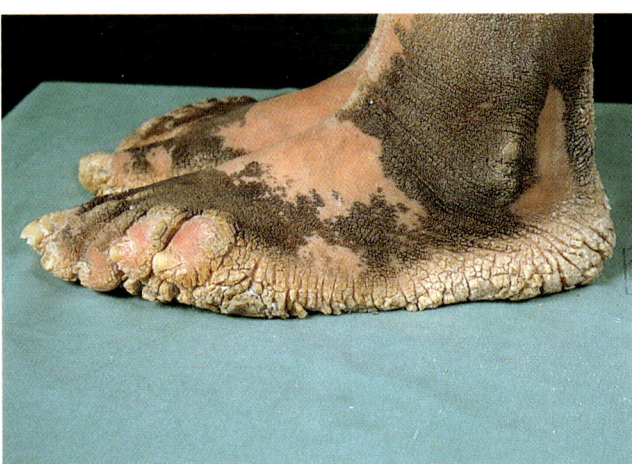

(a)

Figure 3.2(a,b)

Diffuse PPHK: epidermolytic type Vörner. Diffuse hyperkeratosis involves the dorsal aspect of the feet (a) and the soles (b).

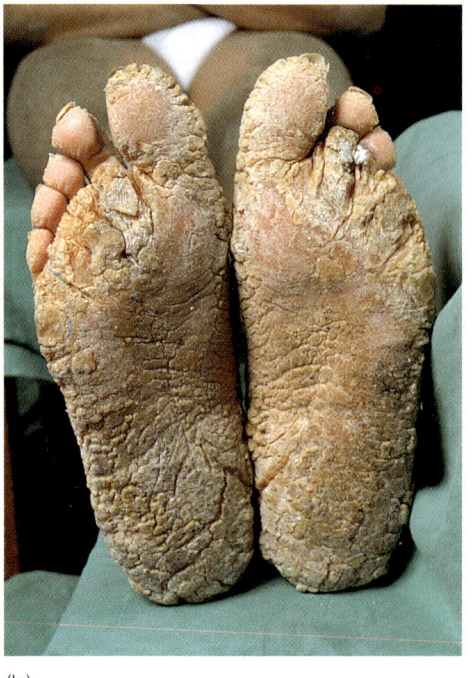

(b)

Diffuse PPHK with associated features

Papillon–Lefèvre syndrome (or PPHK with periodontosis)

This is a recessively inherited disease characterized by a diffuse transgrediens palmoplantar keratosis, psoriasiform lesions on the knees and dorsal aspect of the feet and hyperhidrosis that causes an unpleasant odour. These cutaneous lesions appear between the ages of 1 and 5 years.

Severe gingivostomatitis and periodontitis occur later, with loss of teeth. Patients suffering from the disorder frequently tend to develop pyogenic skin infections. The histologic features of the disease are similar to those observed in Mal de Meleda.

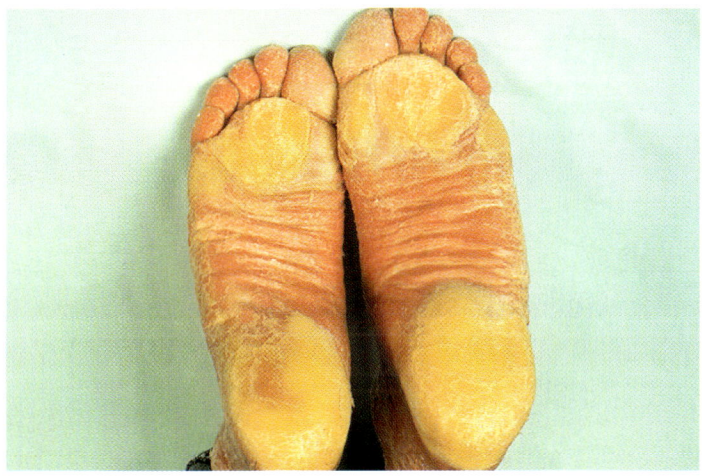

(a)

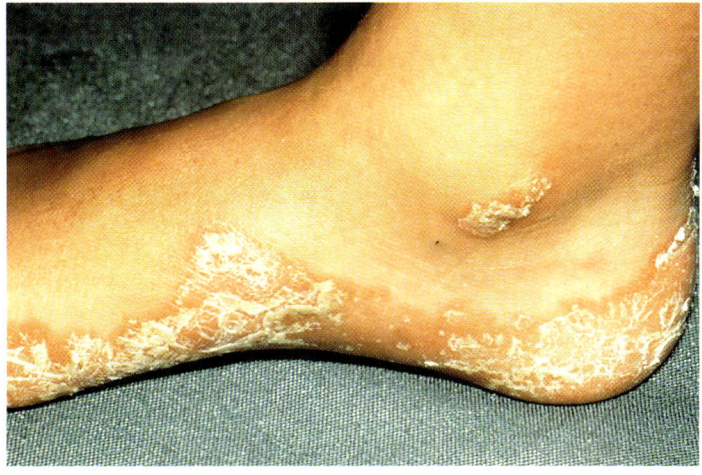

(b)

Figure 3.3(a,b)

Diffuse PPHK Papillon–Lefèvre syndrome. In this example there is a yellowish hyperkeratosis on the balls of the toes and on the heel. Hyperkeratosis is surrounded by erythema. The PPHK is transgrediens because psoriasiform lesions are evident on the back of the feet. The disorder is associated with gingivostomatatis, and hyperhidrosis. (Photograph (b) courtesy of Professor Claudine Blanchet-Bardon.)

PPHK mutilans Vohwinkel

Determined by an autosomal dominant gene, the disorder usually begins in infancy as a diffuse palmoplantar hyperkeratosis that has a honey-comb pattern and a violaceous border. In addition, patients may develop distinctive starfish-shaped keratoses on the dorsal aspect of the lower limbs. The second main clinical feature is constricting fibrous bands that commence in the second decade and that lead progressively to mutilations of the digits. Mutilation of the digits may also occasionally occur in Mal de Meleda, Olmsted syndrome and pachyonychia congenita. Histopathologic findings are a hammock-shaped outline produced by the surface of viable keratinocytes, hypergranulosis and tiny remnants of nuclei in the corneocytes of the stratum corneum.

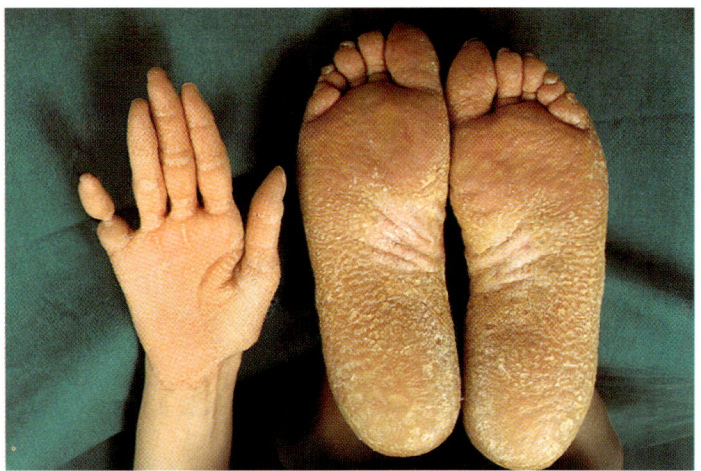

(a)

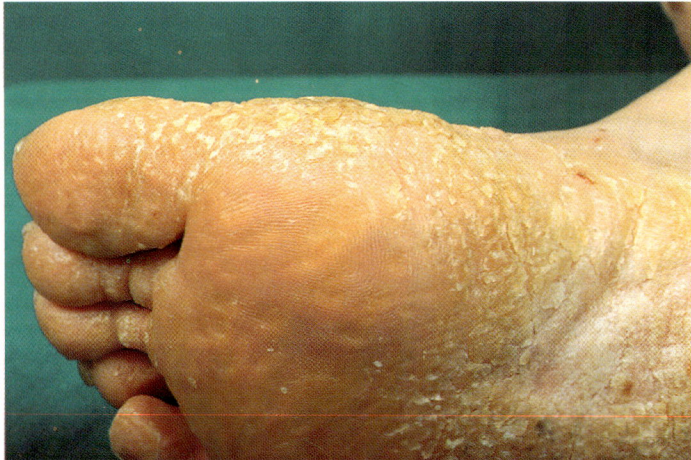

(b)

Figure 3.4(a,b)

Diffuse PPHK with associated features: keratoderma mutilans Vohwinkel. The soles are covered by diffuse hyperkeratosis in a honeycomb pattern. The disorder is associated with the loss of digits as a result of local constrictions (a).

Olmsted syndrome

This is an extremely rare disease that is probably transmitted in an autosomal recessive manner. It is characterized by the unusual association of a well-defined, progressive, transgrediens palmoplantar keratoderma and perioral hyperkeratosis. During childhood, flexion deformities of the digits may lead to constriction phenomena and, progressively, to amputation. The disease is highly disabling because of the severe itching and the painful nature of the keratoderma. This disorder must be differentiated from other mutilating keratodermas, such as Vohwinkel syndrome, Mal de Meleda, pachyonychia congenita. Acrodermatitis enteropathica which can easily be excluded by determining the level of plasma zinc.

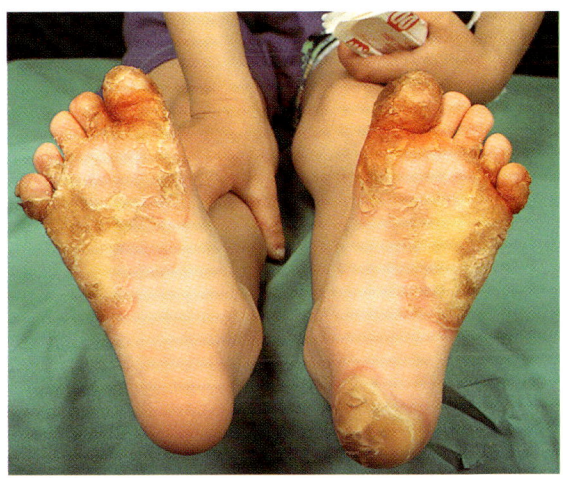

(a)

Figure 3.5(a–c)

Diffuse PPHK: Olmsted syndrome. This disease is characterized by a sharply-demarcated, painful keratoderma that initially involves points of pressure (a). The disease is progressive and transgrediens (b) and is associated with perioral hyperkeratosis, nail dystrophy (c) and deformities of the digits.

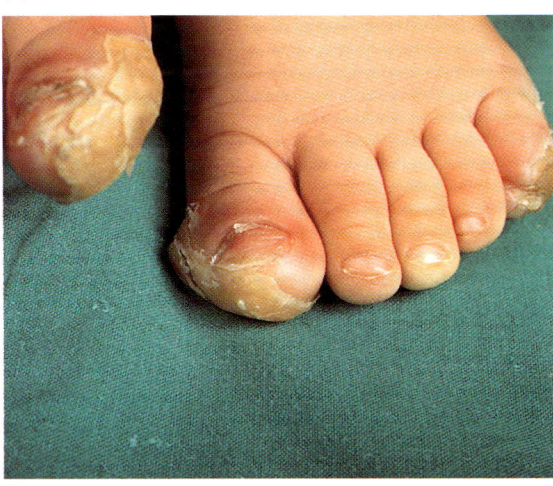

(b)

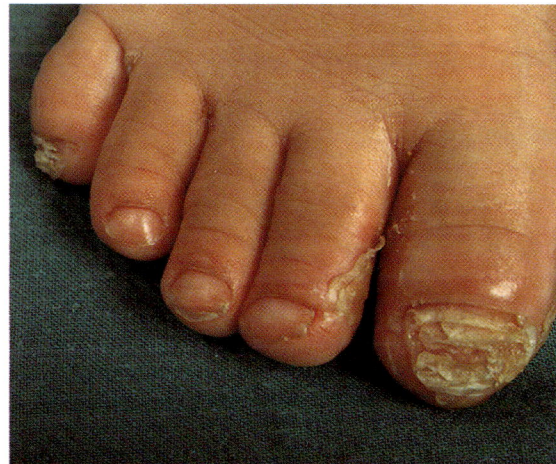

(c)

Hidrotic ectodermal dysplasia (Clouston syndrome)

This disorder consists of dystrophy of the nails, sparsity and defects of the hair, and palmoplantar keratoderma. Hyperkeratosis of the soles has a papillomatous appearance which increases in severity with age. The disease has an autosomal dominant inheritance.

Howell–Evans syndrome (tylosis)

This is an autosomal dominant disorder characterized by a palmoplantar keratoderma associated with carcinoma of the oesophagus. Palmoplantar keratoderma is usually present at birth, whereas oesophageal carcinoma occurs after the age of 40 years.

Focal PPHK

Keratosis Palmoplantaris varians Wachters

Today this term is used to indicate a number of focal PPK inherited via an autosomal dominant trait and that were previously termed Siemens syndrome or Brunauer–Fuchs disease. The plantar lesions usually commence in puberty and consist of insular areas of hyperkeratosis, mainly located on points of pressure. The so-called 'hereditary painful callosities' are a variant of this disorder. The lesions cause pain which is often so intense that walking becomes nearly impossible.

Punctate keratoderma

This is inherited via a regular dominant trait, develops at puberty and is characterized by

numerous yellow to dark brown, round, isolated keratic papules with a central keratic plug. Hyperhidrosis does not occur.

Tyrosinaemia type II (Richner–Hanhart disease) or oculocutaneous tyrosinosis

This is a rare disease determined by an autosomal dominant gene that causes deficiencies in tyrosine aminotransferase, which leads to increased levels of serum tyrosine. The disorder is characterized by the triad of palmoplantar keratoderma, corneal dystrophies (bilateral ulcerative keratitis) and mental retardation. The cutaneous lesions typically consist of painful, discrete, hyperkeratotic plaques on the soles. Bullous lesions and hyperhidrosis may be observed. The discomfort is often proportional to the levels of serum tyrosine.

Pachyonychia congenita

A rare genodermatosis transmitted via an autosomal dominant trait. It is characterized by a combination of ectodermal defects. The main clinical features are hypertrophy and distortion of the nails (100%), palmoplantar hyperkeratosis (60%), leukokeratosis (60%) and follicular keratosis (37%). The palmoplantar keratoderma is symmetrical, non-progressive, nontransgrediens and is mainly located at points of pressure. Hyperhidrosis is common.

Acrokeratoelastoidosis of Costa

This is a marginal keratoderma characterized by rhomboid-shaped papulokeratic lesions distributed along the borders of the hands and feet. Hyperhidrosis is a common feature. The disease is transmitted via an autosomal dominant trait and it usually manifests itself during adolescence.

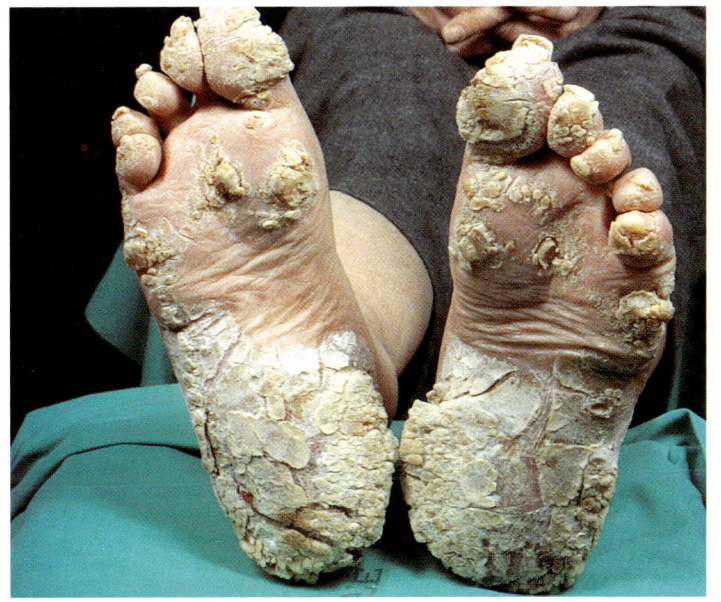

(a)

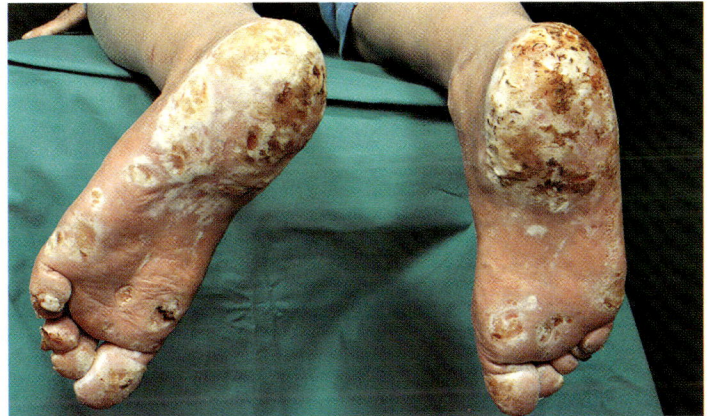

(b)

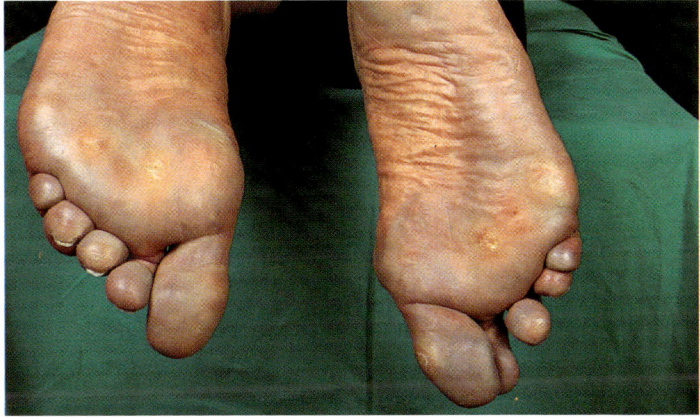

(c)

Figure 3.6(a–c)

Focal PPHK: Wachters syndrome. The lesions consist of insular areas of hyperkeratosis with many fissures, mainly located at points of pressure. The so-called 'hereditary painful callosities' (c) are a variant of this disorder.

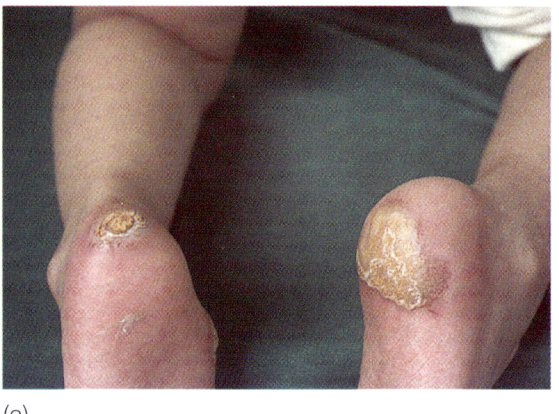

(a)

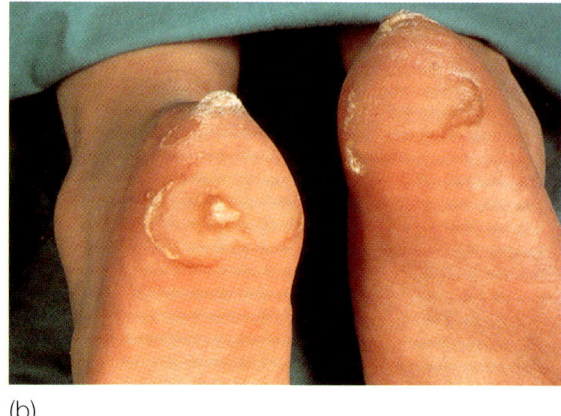

(b)

Figure 3.7(a,b)

Focal PPHK: oculocutaneous tyrosinosis (Richner–Hanhart disease). In this example there are well demarcated, painful, nummular or arcuated hyperkeratotic plaques on the heels. This disorder is due to a deficiency of tyrosine aminotransferase and is characterized by the triad of palmoplantar keratoderma, corneal dystrophies and mental retardation.

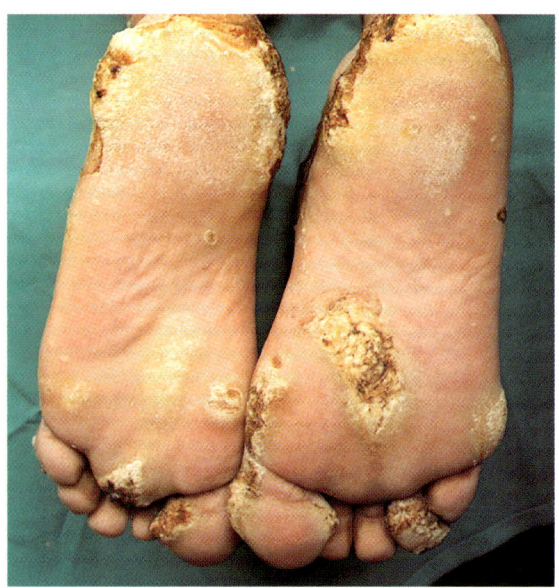

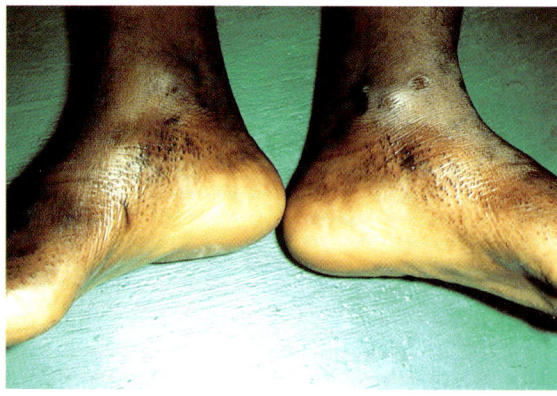

Figure 3.9

Focal PPHK: acrokeratoelastoidosis. Rhomboid-shaped papulokeratic lesions are distributed along the borders of the feet. (Photograph courtesy of Professor Claudine Blanchet-Bardon.)

Figure 3.8

Focal PPHK: pachyonychia congenita. This plantar keratoderma consists of symmetric, not transgradiens areas of hyperkeratosis mainly located at points of pressure. The disorder is characterized by hypertrophy and distortion of the nails and leukokeratosis.

VERRUCOUS EPIDERMAL NAEVI

Verrucous epidermal naevi are permanent, isolated, hamartomatous lesions made up almost exclusively of keratinocytes. They are present at birth in almost 60% of cases but may develop during childhood. Verrucous epidermal naevi can be almost any size and may invade all parts of the body's surface. The surface of most verrucous epidermal naevi is rough, and their colour varies from that of normal skin to red, brown and mousy grey. They are protean in shape and thus may be linear, zosteriform, rectangular and whorled. These naevi may spread beyond the area of original infection. Other abnormalities (cutaneous, systemic or both) may also appear. Verrucous naevi have a wide variety of histological patterns, e.g. epidermolytic hyperkeratosis, focal acantholytic dyskeratosis, verrucous hyperkeratosis parakeratosis and hyperkeratosis.

Clinical features

On the legs and the dorsal aspect of the feet, verrucous naevi tend to be linear, running in a vertical direction. They present as linear, grouped, verrucous, yellowish-brown, keratotic papules that often merge to form a rough-surfaced band.

On the dorsal aspect of the feet, verrucous naevi can also present with the features of a seborrhoeic keratosis or as a large, rough plaque, while on the soles the surface is usually more warty.

Differential diagnosis

Lichen striatus is a self-healing condition (within a few months) consisting of pin-point papules that have either smooth or slightly scaly surfaces.

Linear lichen planus consists of purplish, polygonal, flat-topped papules.

Linear psoriasis comprises whitish scales on the top of reddish plaques.

Inflammatory linear verrucous naevus is an inflammatory pruritic band.

Linear porokeratosis is characterized by an atrophic band with a raised, wall-like border.

The verrucous stage of incontinentia pigmenti is preceded by a vesiculobullous stage.

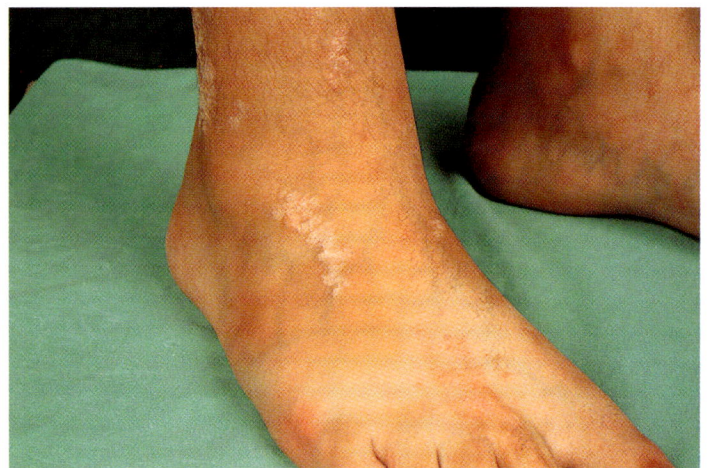

(a)

Figure 3.10(a–c)

Verrucous epidermal naevi. On the dorsal aspect of the feet, verrucous epidermal naevi may present as linear, grouped keratotic papules (a) or as large, rough plaques (b). These lesions are rare on the soles (c) and, when present, are usually warty. The lesions are typically unilateral.

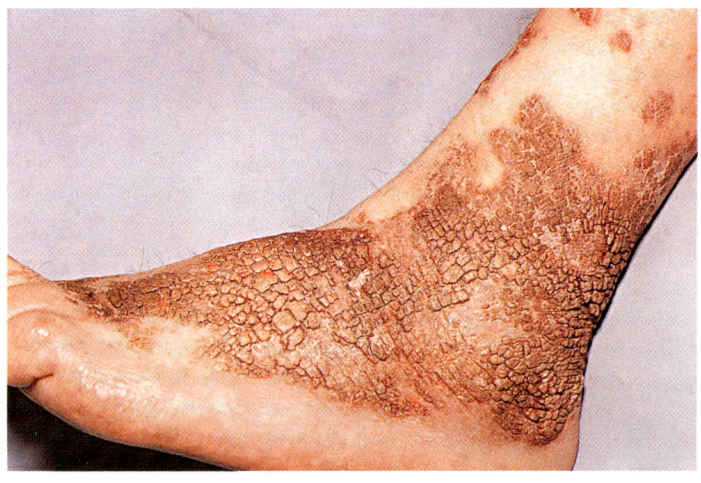

(b)

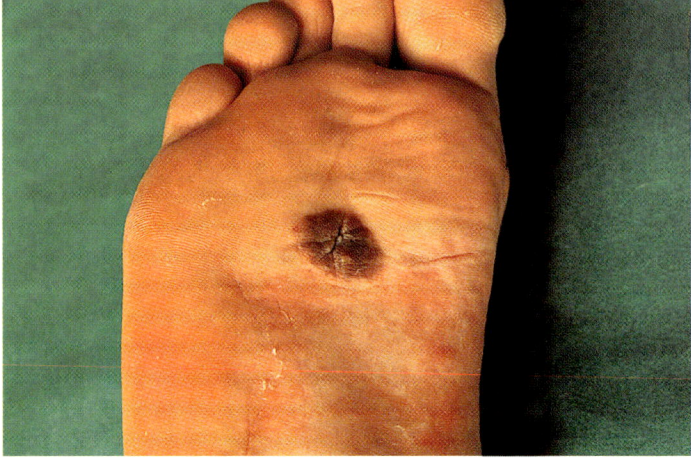

(c)

INFLAMMATORY LINEAR VERRUCOUS NAEVUS

Inflammatory linear verrucous naevus (ILVEN) has a predilection for the lower extremities and is characterized by the following features:

- unilateral lesions that consist of an aggregation of warty papules and that are sharply delineated from normal skin. These coalesce to form plaques or bands, have a clinical resemblance to psoriasis or eczema and are accompanied by intense pruritus;
- an early age of onset (from birth to 5 years);
- resistance to treatment;
- a histological resemblance to either psoriasis or eczema.

Differential diagnosis

Linear verrucous naevi show no signs of inflammation or itching; they have a warty surface.

Lichen striatus is self-healing and comprises either smooth or slightly scaly papules.

Linear lichen planus consists of purplish, polygonal, flat-topped papules.

Linear psoriasis is usually associated with other psoriatic lesions and is asymptomatic.

Linear neurodermatitis occurs in adults; it usually responds promptly to treatment.

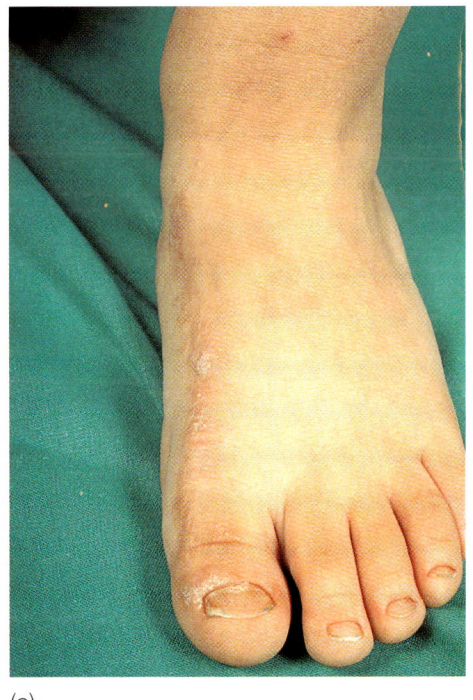

(a)

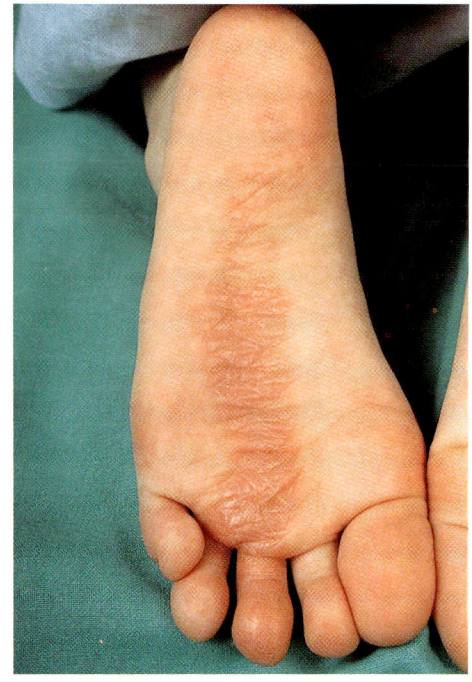

(b)

Figure 3.11(a,b)

Inflammatory linear verrucous naevi. These unilateral, pruritic bands consist of an aggregation of papules that are sharply delineated from normal skin. On the back of the foot the lesions are warty (a) but smooth on the sole (b).

POROKERATOSIS

Porokeratosis is a rare, chronic, progressive, asymptomatic keratoatrophoderma of different clinical forms that are histologically characterized by columns of parakeratosis termed 'cornoid lamellae'.

Five clinical variants have been described: the classic plaque porokeratosis of Mibelli, disseminated superficial porokeratosis, disseminated superficial actinic porokeratosis, porokeratosis punctata palmaris and plantaris, and linear porokeratosis.

In all these forms of porokeratosis, the primary lesion is a small, hyperkeratotic papule that enlarges gradually to form a plaque or a band with a raised, wall-like border that resembles a dike. It also has an atrophic, depressed centre.

The disease usually occurs during childhood and may undergo malignant change.

Clinical features

On the feet, the most common forms are porokeratosis punctata and linear porokeratosis. Porokeratosis punctata presents on the soles as numerous, 1–2 mm, seed-like keratotic plugs arising from rimmed crypts. In linear porokeratosis the lesion assumes a zosteriform unilateral distribution with a prominent, raised border.

Differential diagnosis

The raised, wall-like borders and the depressed atrophic centre are the distinctive clinical features of these diseases. Histologically they are characterized by the presence of columns of parakeratosis (cornoid lamellae). These features make porokeratoses readily identifiable. The punctate variant must be differentiated from naevoid basal-cell carcinoma syndrome, Darier's disease and punctate keratoderma, while the linear variant needs differentiation from linear verrucous epidermal naevus, linear psoriasis, linear lichen planus and lichen striatus.

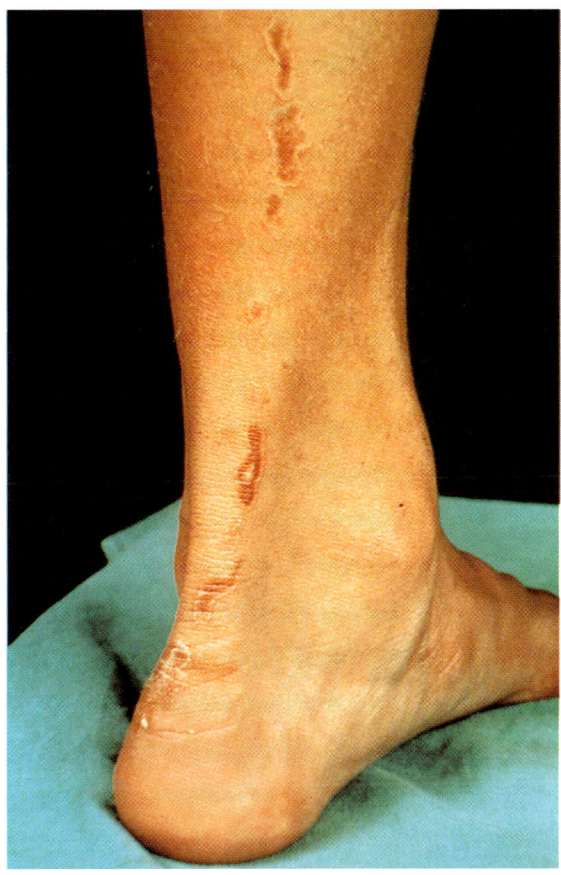

(a)

Figure 3.12(a,b)

Linear porokeratosis. The lesions consist of a band (a) or elongated plaque (b) with a raised, wall–like border that resembles a dike. This has an atrophic, depressed centre.

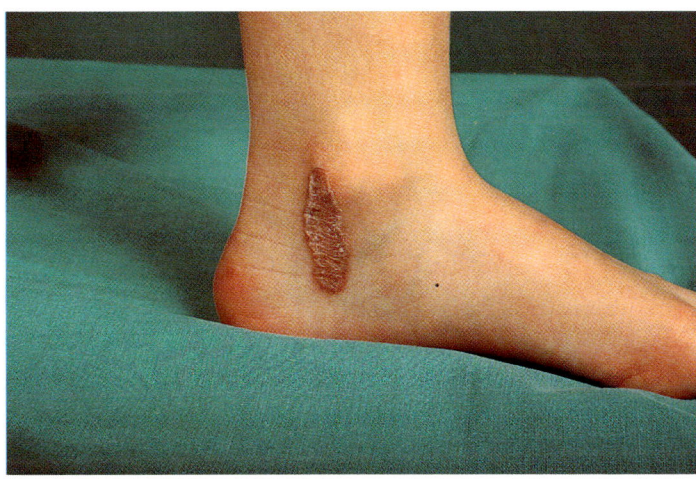

(b)

PITYRIASIS RUBRA PILARIS

Pityriasis rubra pilaris (PRP) is a keratinization disorder of unknown aetiology characterized by follicular plugging (mainly involving the elbows and knees), perifollicular erythema, cephalic rash and palmoplantar hyperkeratosis.

The age of onset is bimodal, with peaks during the first and fifth decades. It is possible to distinguish two adult forms (classic and atypical) and three juvenile forms (classic, localized and atypical). The disease is usually self-healing, but the course may vary from a few months to several years. Histologically the disease is characterized by a chess-board pattern of alternating ortho- and parakeratosis within a thickened horny layer.

Clinical features

Follicular keratotic papules, surrounded by a classic yellow-orange ring, are located on the dorsal aspect of the feet. It also presents with a sharply demarcated, diffuse, plantar keratoderma that has a characteristic salmon colour. Occasionally, oedema may be observed. The Achilles tendons are frequently involved. An onychodystrophy may occur in the form of longitudinal striae. Pruritus is usually absent.

Differential diagnosis

Psoriasis: the salmon colour usually seen in PRP is absent.

Keratosis pilaris: the keratotic lesions are extremely small and not erythematous; the plantar aspect is usually spared.

Inherited and acquired palmoplantar keratodermas: the salmon colour is absent.

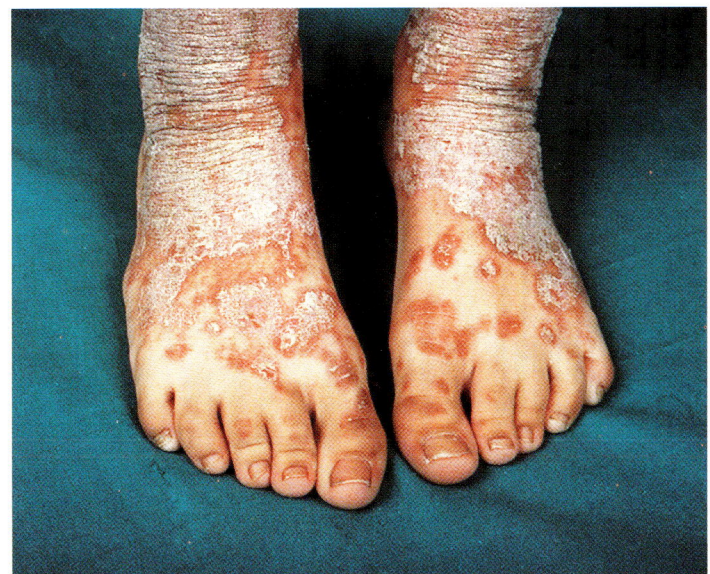

Figure 3.13

Pityriasis rubra pilaris. Plaques covered by whitish scales and surrounded by a yellow-orange halo are distributed symmetrically on the dorsal aspect of the feet.

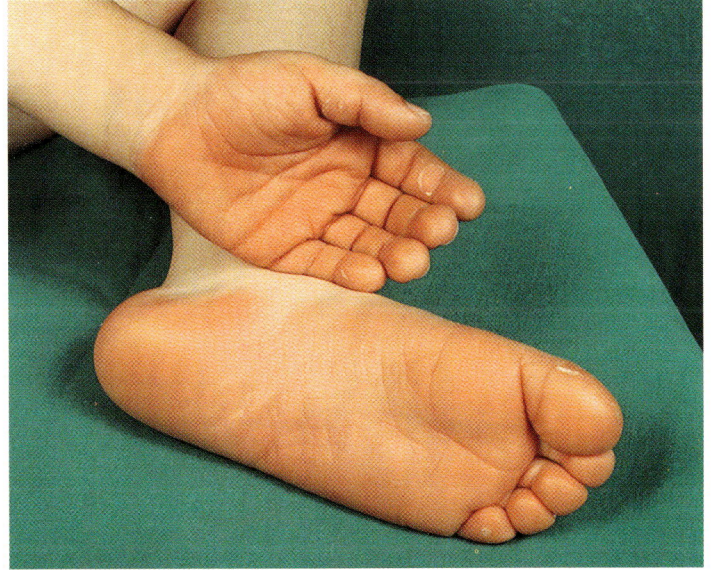

Figure 3.14

Pityriasis rubra pilaris. This example shows a sharply demarcated, palmoplantar keratoderma of the typical salmon colour.

DARIER'S DISEASE

Darier's disease is a dominantly inherited skin disease characterized clinically by grey-brown, keratic, mostly non-follicular papules located predominantly on the 'seborrhoeic' areas (face, auricles, neck, chest and mid-line of the back). Hand involvement has been observed in 90% of patients, while the feet are involved in only about 30% of cases. The nails are commonly affected; fragility and longitudinal splits are typical findings. The disorder tends to disappear from the age of 5 years through the teenage years.

Acral Darier's disease is clinically identical to so-called acrokeratosis verruciformis. Focal acantholytic dyskeratosis is the distinctive histologic feature.

Clinical features

Three main features may be present on the feet:

- flat, wart-like papules resembling acrokeratosis verruciformis lesions may be present on the backs of the feet and toes. These lesions are usually bilaterally located;
- plantar pits and keratotic papules may be observed in about 30% of patients;
- a diffuse hyperkeratosis of the soles is seen in about 10% of patients.

The toenails may be involved, but less often and less severely than the fingernails.

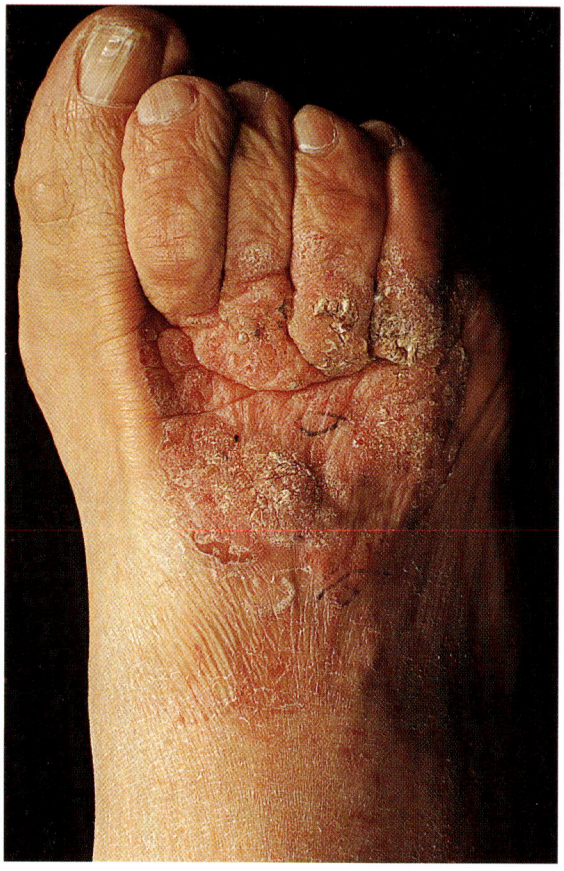

Figure 3.15
Darier's disease. This plaque is the result of the agglomeration wart-like papules.

Differential diagnosis

The presence of the disorder's typical lesions on seborrhoeic areas and on the nails permits easy differentiation of the wart-like papules from the wart lesions of epidermodysplasia verruciformis and the papules of lichen planus.

The pits on the soles seen in naevoid basal-cell carcinoma are frequently surrounded by a thin rim of erythema, and are associated with numerous basal-cell carcinomas, jaw cysts, skeletal anomalies and ectopic calcifications.

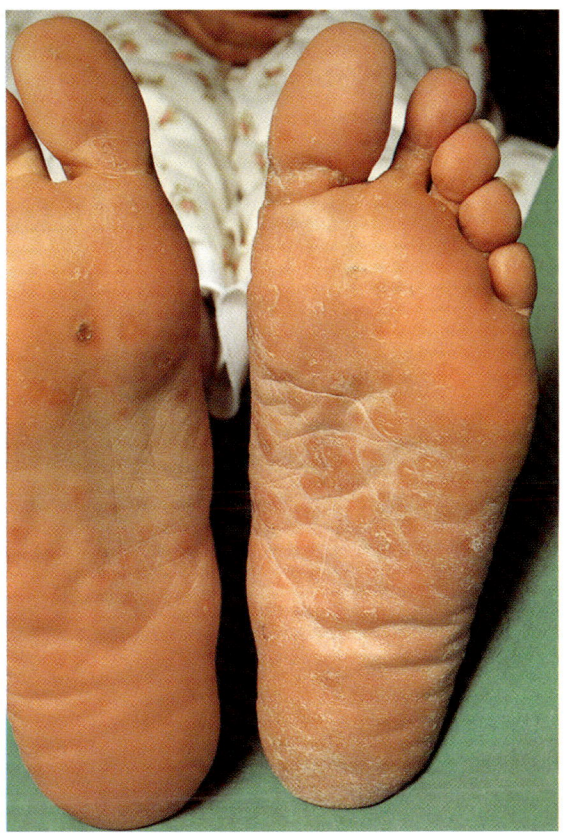

(a)

Figure 3.16(a,b)

Darier's disease. On the soles, this disorder may occur as keratotic papules (a) or as diffuse hyperkeratosis (b). A small number of isolated pits may be seen on the plantar aspect of the toes (b).

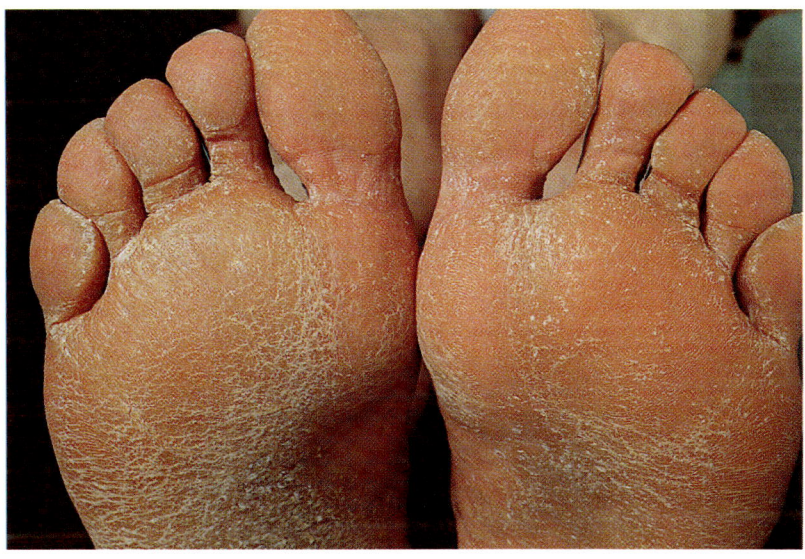

(b)

EPIDERMODYSPLASIA VERRUCIFORMIS

Epidermodysplasia verruciformis (EV) is a rare disease that is transmitted via an autosomal recessive gene. It is characterized by a generalized, cutaneous infection with human papilloma virus; depressed, cell-mediated immunity; and a propensity (in 30% of cases) for the cutaneous lesions to convert malignant to basal-cell or squamous cell carcinoma in predominantly sun-exposed areas of the body.

Three main types of skin lesion may be present: flat warts, mostly located on the extremities and the face; pityresis versicolor like-plaques preferentially involving the trunk; and vegetating, brown seborrhoeic wart-like lesions observed on the scalp and face. The disease usually occurs in childhood.

Clinical features

In patients with EV, plane warts are readily seen on the backs of the feet. On the soles, three types of lesion have been observed: common warts, pits and vegetating plaques.

Differential diagnosis

The warty lesions of EV located on the backs of the hands and feet are very similar to those of acrokeratosis verruciformis but, in this disease, histologically there are no vacuolated cells in the upper layers of the epidermis. In lichen planus the papules are pink, pruritic and may involve the mucous membranes. The pits, rarely present on the soles, may be differentiated from those seen in Darier's disease and in basal cell naevus only histologically.

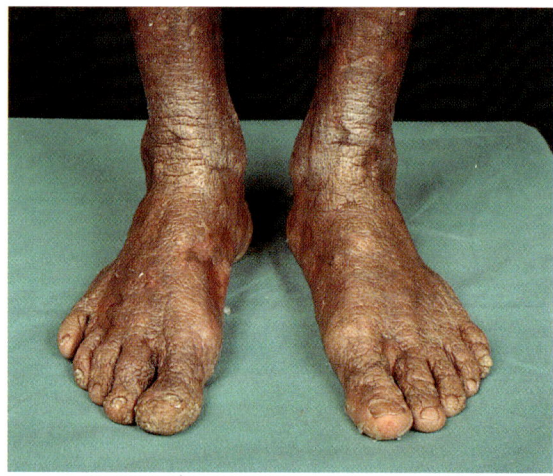

(a)

Figure 3.17(a,b)
Epidermodysplasia verruciformis. In this patient, plane warts are present on the back of the feet (a), while a vegetating plaque is located on the sole (b).

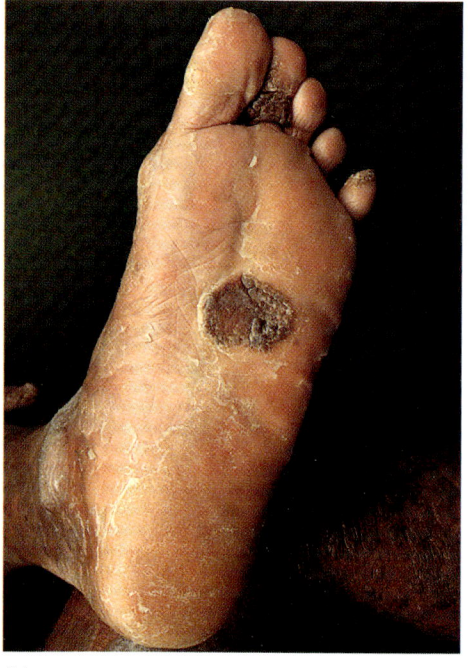

(b)

HEREDITARY EPIDERMOLYSIS BULLOSA

Epidermolysis bullosa (EB) is a term encompassing a wide spectrum of hereditary skin disorders characterized by a tendency to form blisters even after minor mechanical trauma. These disorders may subdivide (by electron microscopy) into three major forms – epidermolytic, junctional and dermolytic – according to where the plane of separation of blisters is perceived to have occurred. In the epidermolytic forms blisters are intraepidermal, in the junctional forms blisters are in the lamina lucida and in the dermatolytic forms blisters are beneath the lamina densa. At least 18 subtypes of EB have been recognized to date. In this section only those that have major involvement with the feet will be discussed.

Epidermolysis bullosa simplex

EB simplex Köbner

This disease is inherited via an autosomal dominant trait and is usually present at birth. The blisters are widespread but have predilection for the hands and feet. The blisters worsen in summer and heal spontaneously without scarring. The nails are unaffected.

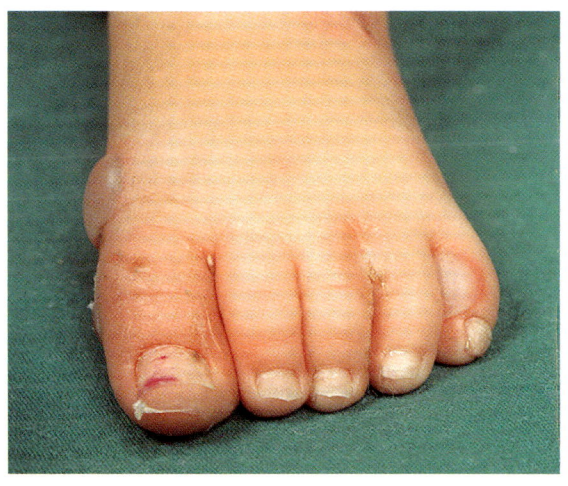

(a)

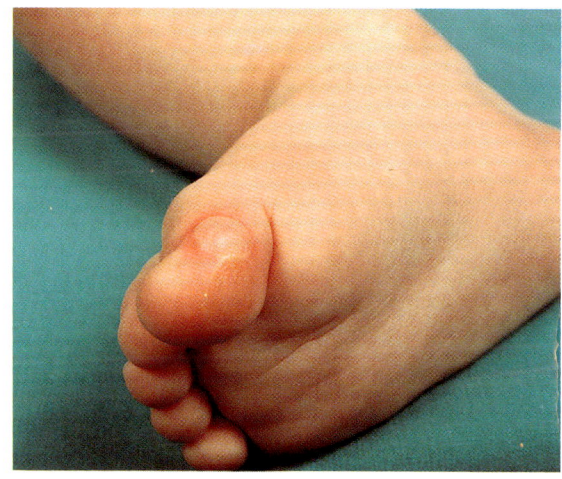

(b)

Figure 3.18(a,b)
Epidermolytic epidermolysis bullosa. Blisters are present at birth, have a predilection for the feet, worsen in summer and heal spontaneously without scarring. The nails are normal.

EB simplex localisata Weber–Cockayne

This variant is inherited via an autosomal dominant trait. Onset is usually during the first or second year or life, but it may occur at a later age. Recurrent bullae develop on the hands and feet. Hyperhidrosis is a complication. The mucosa and nails are spared.

EB herpetiformis Dowling–Meara

This condition is inherited via a dominant trait. It appears at birth with severe generalized blistering. The hands and feet are severely affected. The blisters may house haemorrhagic contents, are surrounded by rims of redness and are distributed in a herpetiform pattern. The blisters heal without scarring, but milia formation may occur. The nails are often involved but they usually heal normally. A palmoplantar hyperkeratosis may be present. After the age of 7 years, progressive improvement is usual.

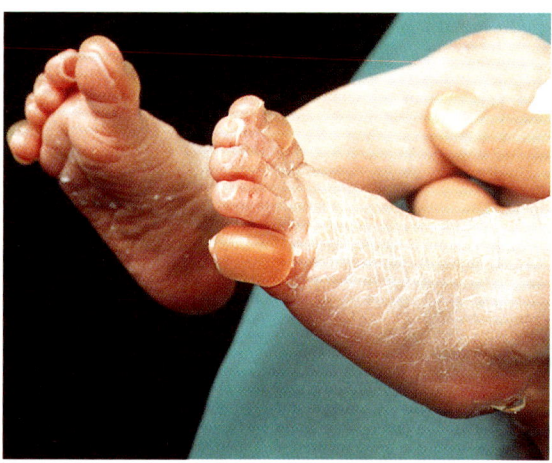

Figure 3.19
Epidermolytic epidermolysis bullosa: EB simplex localisata Weber–Cockayne. In this localized form, blisters are confined to a single anatomic site and heal without scars.

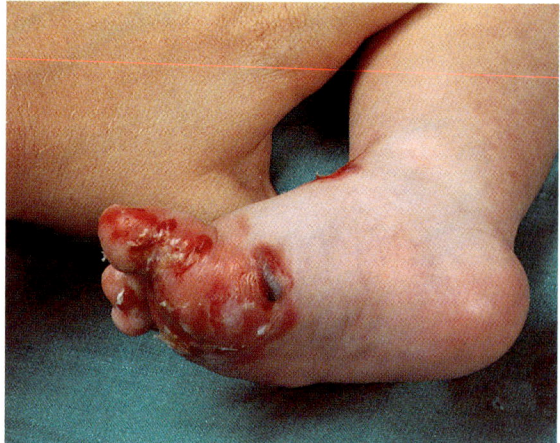

(a)

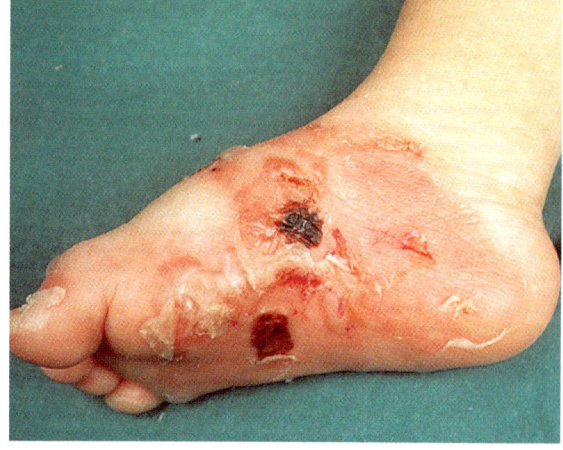

(b)

Figure 3.20(a,b)
Epidermolytic epidermolysis bullosa: FR herpetiformis Dowling–Meara. In this condition there is a generalized blistering, but the hands and feet are the sites most commonly affected. The blisters are surrounded by a rim of redness, are distributed in a herpetiform pattern and may be haemorrhagic.

Junctional epidermolysis bullosa

This group of diseases are inherited in an autosomal recessive manner. Manifestations vary from mild involvement (EB atrophica generalizata mitis, EB atrophicans inversa, EB atrophicans localisata) to a life-threatening form (EB atrophicans letalis Herlitz). These all heal without scarring but atrophy may develop with time. In these forms the feet are relatively spared, their involvement only being evident in EB atrophicans localisata. In this disorder blisters occur primarily on the soles and lower extremities, commencing at the age of 5 years. Blisters develop spontaneously or post-traumatically, mainly during the summer. Plantar blisters are followed by painful erosions.

Dystrophic epidermolysis bullosa

Localized dominant dystrophic EB Cockayne–Touraine

Blisters secondary to trauma develop only on the extremities, especially the dorsal aspect of the hands and feet. Healing occurs with scarring and milia. The nails are often dystrophic. The mucous membranes are spared. Onset is in infancy or early childhood.

Widespread dominant dystrophic EB Pasini

Usually present at birth. It is characterized by a generalized eruption of blisters primarily involving the extremities. Blisters leave atrophic scars and milia. The major distinguishing feature of this disorder is the spontaneous appearance during puberty of ivory papules on the trunk that resemble small scars.

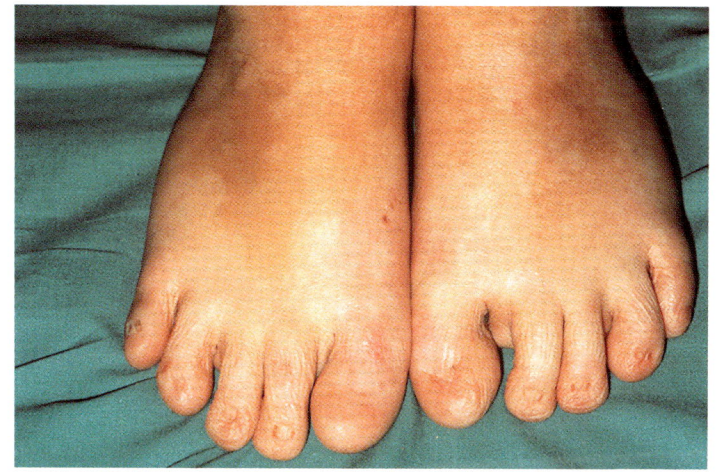

Figure 3.21
Dystrophic epidermolysis bullosa: localized dominant EB dystrophica Cockayne–Touraine. In this disorder, blisters secondary to trauma develop on the extremities. These heal with scars. The nails are dystrophic.

Recessive dystrophic EB Hallopeau–Siemens

Appears at birth with widespread blisters and oral involvement. Healing occurs slowly, with atrophy scars and milia. The frequent recurrence of the blisters causes cicatricial fusion of the fingers and toes (syndactyly). A mitten-like deformity of the hands and feet may develop. Nails are dystrophic or disappear. Mucosal involvement appears early and may be severe. Teeth are usually malformed.

Recessive inverse EB

Affects the inguinal and axillary folds, the neck and the lumber region. The feet are usually spared.

Bart's syndrome

A congenital, localized absence of skin (aplasia cutis) that affects the lower extremities. It is associated with the dominant and recessive type of EB dystrophica, as well as with the Herlitz type of junctional EB.

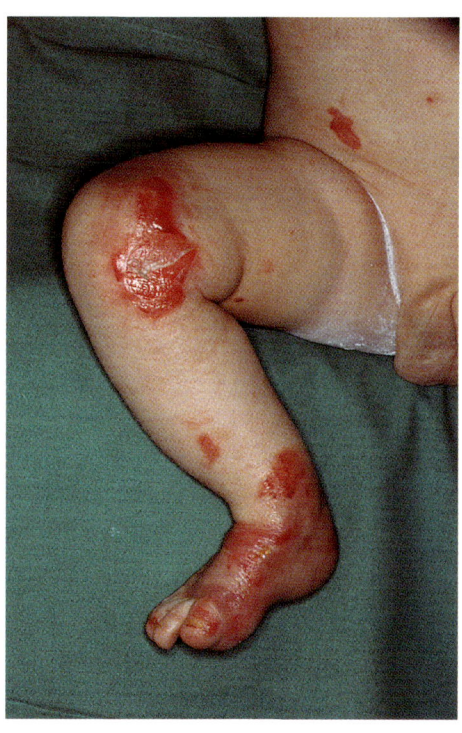

(a)

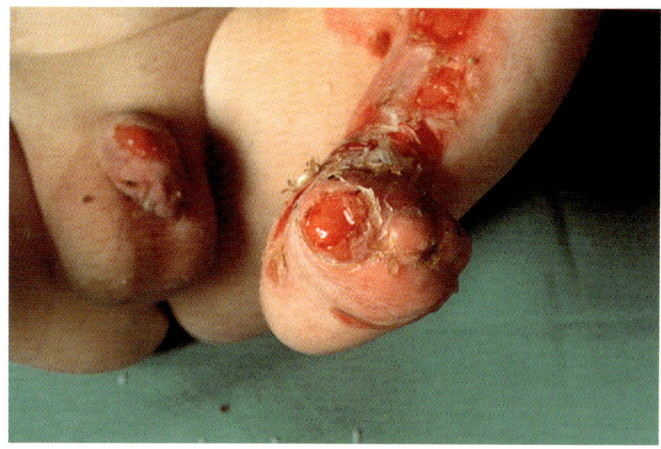

(b)

Figure 3.22(a,b)

Dystrophic epidermolysis bullosa: recessive EB dystrophica Hallopeau–Siemens. These extensive areas of de-epithelization are present at birth and heal slowly with atrophic scars and milia. Repeated subepidermal blisters may cause cicatricial fusion of the toes.

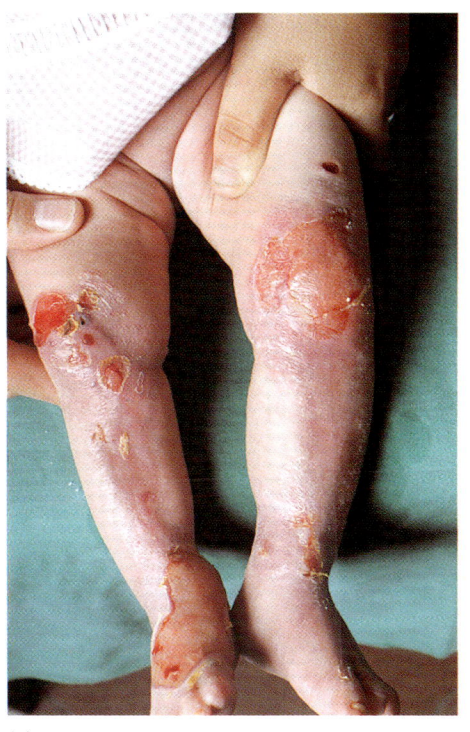

(a)

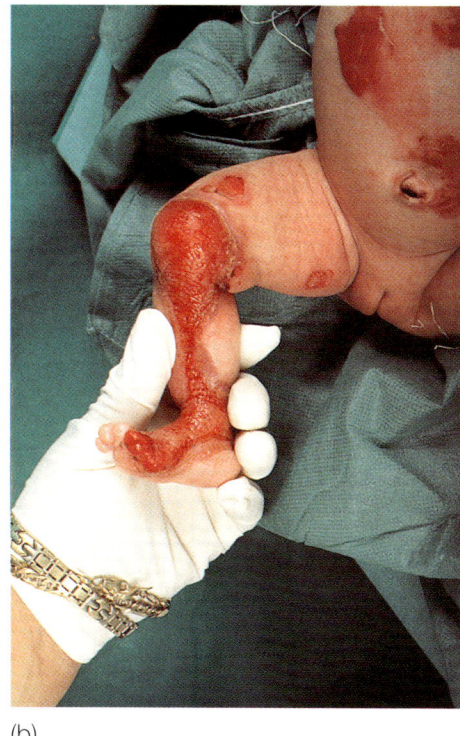

(b)

Figure 3.23(a,b)

Dystrophic epidermolysis bullosa: Bart's syndrome. In this disorder there is a congenital localized absence of skin (aplasia cutis) that affects the lower extremities. The disorder is associated with lesions of EB dystrophica.

INCONTINENTIA PIGMENTI

Incontinentia pigmenti is a rare, X-linked, dominant genodermatosis typically characterized by growing cutaneous lesions, that are arranged in whorls and streaks along Blaschko's lines. The disease is present at birth or shortly thereafter. Classically, the cutaneous lesions develop in four stages. In the first stage, there is a linear, erythemato-vesicular and bullous eruption (erythematous bullous stage). After a few weeks these are replaced by verrucous lesions (verrucous stage). As the verrucous lesions involute, whorled and linear zones of hyperpigmentation appear (pigmentary stage), which are more evident on the trunk. These lesions usually fade gradually during adolescence. The fourth stage, if present, is characterized by streaky hypopigmentation and atrophy, mainly on the lower extremities. This disease is frequently associated with dental, ocular and central nervous system anomalies.

Clinical features

On the dorsal aspect of the feet, the lesions follow Blascko's lines. At this site, verrucous keratic lesions are readily seen. Painful subungual keratotic tumours may appear after puberty.

Differential diagnosis

The erythematous and vesiculo-bullous lesions in newborn babies are easily differentiated from epidermolysis bullosa, bullous lamellar ichthyosis and bullous impetigo because none of these disorders follow Blaschko's lines.

Epidermal naevi are ruled out because the verrucous lesions are not preceded by a vesiculo-bullous stage. Lichen striatus follows Blaschko's lines but disappears in a few months. Hyperpigmented lesions must be differentiated from linear naevoid hypermelanosis; this disorder is not preceded by inflammatory stages.

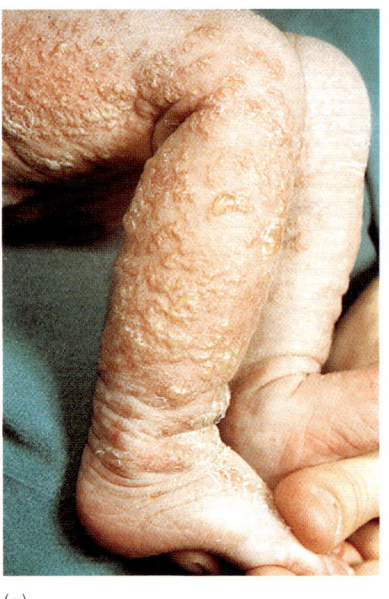

(a)

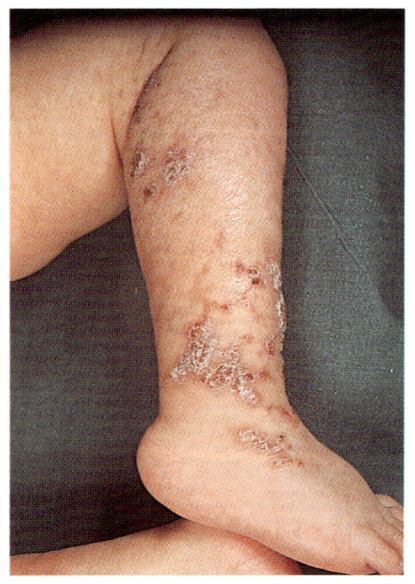

(b)

Figure 3.24(a,b)

Incontinentia pigmenti. In the erythematous bullous stage (a), the lesions consist of vesicles on skin-coloured or reddish-brown base merging in a reticulated fashion. In the verrucous stage (b) the lesions are papulokeratic.

ACRODERMATITIS ENTEROPATHICA

Acrodermatitis enteropathica is a rare, autosomal recessive disease caused by zinc deficiency. It is characterized by the triad of perioral and acral dermatitis, diarrhoea and alopecia. Initially, the skin lesions are eczematoid, with crops of vesicles and pustules; subsequently they become psoriasiform, with a reddish plaque covered in scales and crusts. These signs are evident by the time the infant has been weaned from maternal milk. A low serum level of zinc (less than 500 mg/day) is a cardinal finding.

Histopathologically, there is a marked ballooning of keratinocytes in the upper part of the epidermis as well as parakeratosis.

Clinical features

On the feet the skin lesions are usually psoriasiform and mainly involve the heels and toes. Nail changes are frequent and consist of onychodystrophy, onycholysis and paronychia.

Differential diagnosis

Skin lesions of psoriasis are usually more scaly, have a different location and are not accompanied by diarrhoea and alopecia. In candidiasis there is no zinc deficiency. Epidermolysis bullosa comprises blisters, which are not a feature of acrodermatitis enteropathica.

In adults, lesions indistinguishable from those of acrodermatitis enteropathica may be observed in acquired zinc deficiency disorders arising as a consequence of Crohn's disease, malabsorption syndromes, glucagonoma syndrome, bowel bypass syndrome and systemic malignancies.

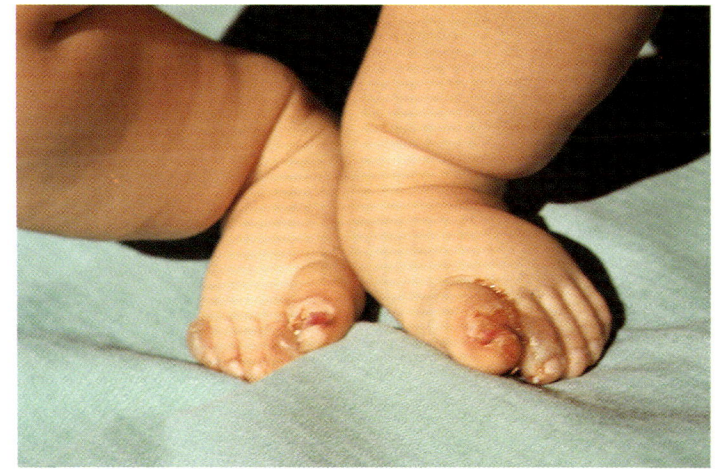

Figure 3.25

Acrodermatitis enteropathica. In this patient, blisters and scales have affected the toes. The big toes on both feet display paronychia and onychodystrophy.

4 Infectious and parasitic disorders

STAPHYLOCOCCAL SCALDED-SKIN SYNDROME
ERYSIPELAS
ECTHYMA
GRAM-NEGATIVE INFECTIONS
CAT-SCRATCH DISEASE
TUBERCULOSIS
SYPHILIS
TINEA PEDIS
CANDIDIASIS
SPOROTRICHOSIS
CHROMOBLASTOMYCOSIS
MYCETOMAS
PRIMARY HERPES SIMPLEX
WARTS
HAND-FOOT-AND-MOUTH DISEASE
PAPULAR-PURPURIC 'GLOVES AND SOCKS' SYNDROME
CUTANEOUS LARVA MIGRANS
FILARIASIS
FLEA INFESTATIONS
TUNGIASIS
SCABIES
JELLYFISH INFESTATIONS

STAPHYLOCOCCAL SCALDED-SKIN SYNDROME

Staphylococcal scalded-skin syndrome (SSSS) is an acute and severe disorder caused by two staphylococcal exotoxins. These toxins, called A and B, are produced mainly by *Staphylococcus aureus* of phage group II, type 71.

The syndrome is more frequent in neonates and infants.

Clinical features

SSSS is characterized initially by a diffuse or generalized erythematous, macular (scarlatiniform) rash, sometimes with scattered vesicles and/or blisters. Nikolsky's sign is usually positive. This phase is followed by a true epidermolysis, which produces a wrinkling of the skin; this becomes erythematous and may be removed easily. The underlying surface appears intensely red and moist. Mucous membranes are rarely involved. Fever, general malaise and lymphadenopathy are frequent.

Differential diagnosis

Bacteria responsible for SSSS are obtained neither from sites of sloughing skin, nor from vesicles or blisters. They must be searched for at sites of primary colonization (e.g. external ear canal, oropharynx, tonsils, nares and umbilical stump).

Toxic epidermal necrolysis is very often drug-induced and much commoner in adults. The mucous membranes are always involved.

Toxic shock syndrome is much commoner in females during the third decade of life.

Kawasaki's syndrome is characterized by three clinical phases, in which involvement of the mucous membranes, heart, joints and lymph nodes is characteristic.

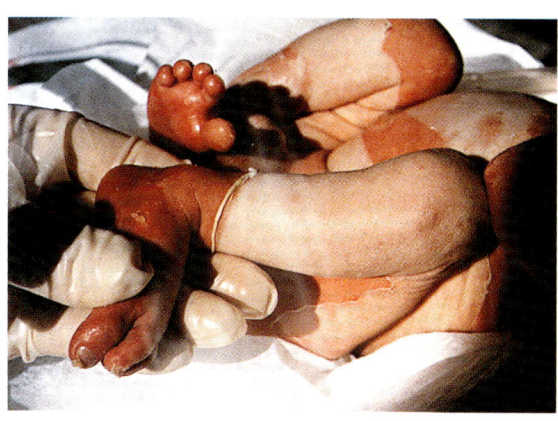

Figure 4.1
Staphylococcal scalded-skin syndrome. The epidermis can be easily removed.

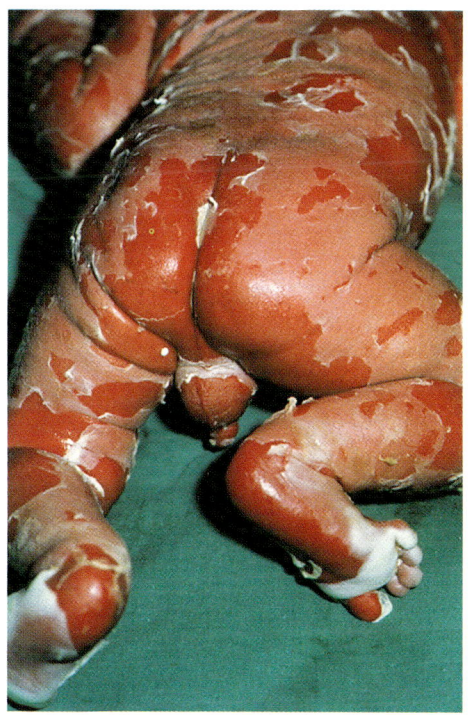

Figure 4.2
Staphylococcal scalded-skin syndrome. The surface under the epidermis appears intensely red and moist.

ERYSIPELAS

Erysipelas is a bacterial disease of the dermis and subcutaneous tissue caused, in most cases, by group A β-haemolytic *Streptococcus pyogenes*. However, *Staphylococcus aureus* is emerging as an aetiological agent. Currently, these bacteria are responsible for the disease in more than 30% of patients. Local predisposing factors are venous insufficiency, and venous and post-traumatic ulcers. The legs are affected in 85–90% of patients. Erysipelas is usually preceded by general malaise, asthenia, fever and chills. These symptoms, as well as lymphangitis and lymphadenitis, may accompany the skin manifestations.

Clinical features

Erysipelas is uncommon on the feet. It is characterized by erythematous swelling, very often of several centimetres in diameter; bright red in colour and with sharply defined and elevated borders. The skin is hot, tender and parenchymatously-hard in consistency. Inside the lesions, vesicles, bullae, pustules, erosions and ulcers may develop.

Recurrent erysipelas induces the development of elephantiasis nostra streptogenes, a chronic form of oedema and lymphoedema that occurs as a result of lymphatic subocclusion and occlusion.

Differential diagnosis

Gram's stain and culture of material obtained from open lesions may sometimes prove positive for bacteria.

Measurement of serum ASOT may be helpful. Differential diagnosis includes other bacterial diseases (e.g. abscess, erysipeloid and necrotizing fasciitis).

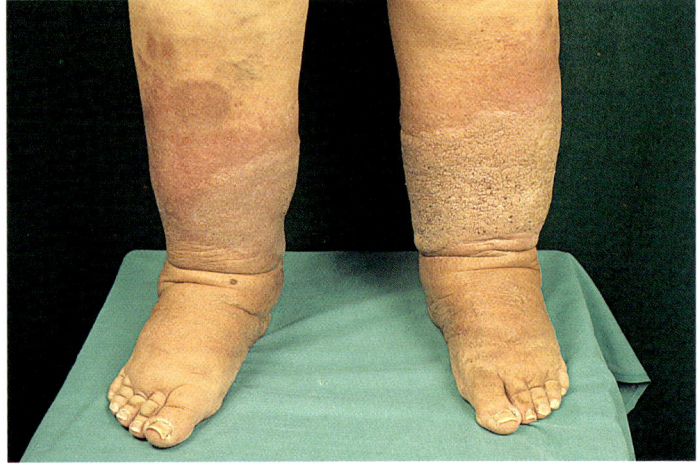

Figure 4.3
Elephantiasis. Chronic oedema and lymphoedema following recurrent episodes of erysipelas.

ECTHYMA

Ecthyma is a disease caused by cocci. *Staphylococcus aureus* and group A β-haemolytic *Streptococcus pyogenes* are most commonly involved. Mixed infections caused by both bacteria are not uncommon. Diabetes, immunosuppression, alcoholism and drug abuse are considered predisposing factors.

The buttocks, thighs, legs and back of the feet are the most frequent locations.

Clinical features

The lesions of ecthyma are generally multiple and discrete. The primary lesion may be a mildly inflammatory vesicle, bulla or pustule. However, in most cases, patients present with a thick adherent crust. Removal of the crust reveals a round or oval, more or less deep ulcer, with a base covered by purulent exudate and necrotic material. The ulcer may be surrounded by an erythematous halo. The patient usually complains of pain. Regional lympadenopathy may be present.

Differential diagnosis

Gram's stain and culture show, respectively, the presence of cocci and the growth of micro-organisms responsible for the disease.

Other primary bacterial infections (e.g. impetigo) of the skin must be taken into consideration in differential diagnosis. Moreover, numerous cutaneous diseases may undergo secondary bacterial superinfections.

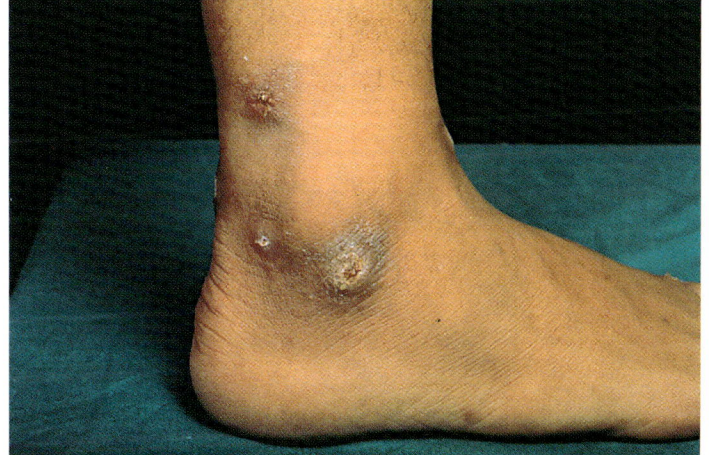

Figure 4.4
Ecthyma. A thick and adherent crust covers the underlying ulcer.

GRAM-NEGATIVE INFECTIONS

Gram-negative infections are caused by different aetiological agents, although *Pseudomonas aeruginosa* is the most frequent. Amongst other agents, *Serratia marcescens* and *Escherichia coli* may be involved. Furthermore, mixed infections as a consequence of these and other bacteria – both Gram-negative and Gram-positive – are not uncommon.

Clinical manifestations are similar, despite the fact that different bacteria may be responsible for the infection.

Clinical features

Gram-negative infections occur in the interdigital spaces. The skin appears macerated and erythematous, with linear erosions and rhagades. The lesions are circumscribed by a macerated, whitish collarette. With time, the dorsal aspect of the feet, and the soles, may also become affected. When *Pseudomonas aeruginosa* is the aetiological agent, a characteristic greenish exudate oozes from the lesions.

The disease is usually tender.

Differential diagnosis

Gram's stain and culture of the exudate reveal, respectively, the presence and the growth of bacteria, in particular *Pseudomonas aeruginosa*.

The negativity of Wood's lamp, and direct and cultural mycological examinations, allow differentiation from tinea pedis.

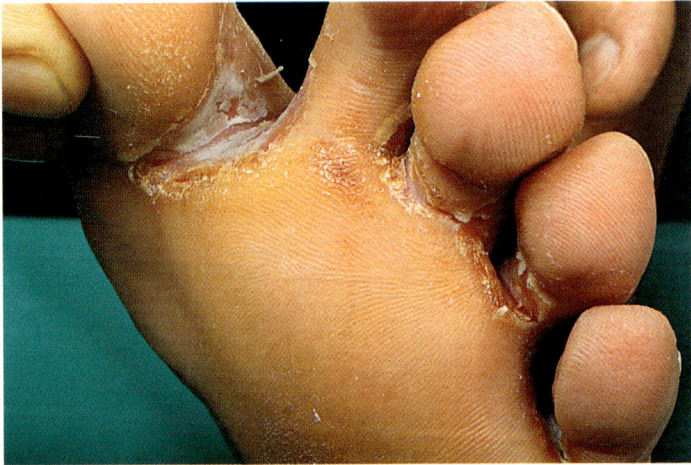

Figures 4.5 and 4.6
Gram-negative infections. A whitish collarette circumscribes an erosive-ulcerative lesion.

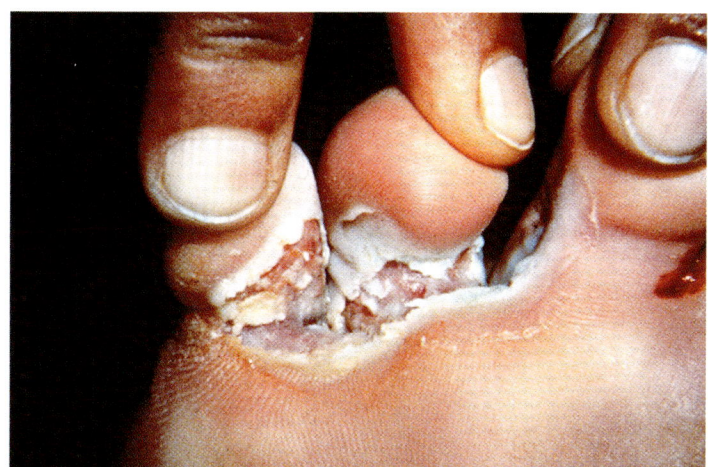

Figure 4.6

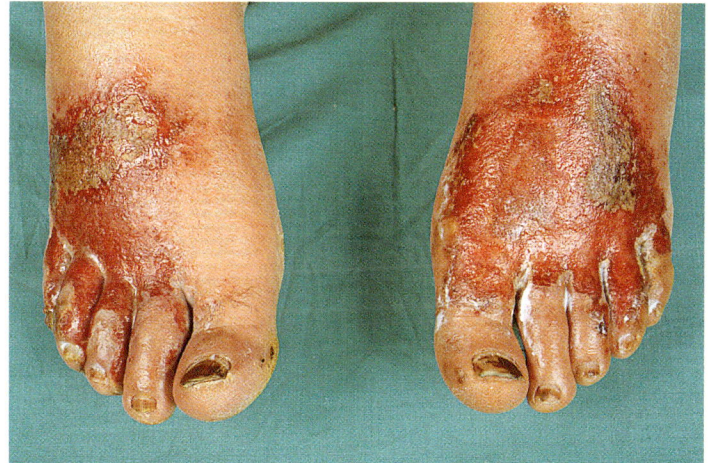

Figure 4.7
Gram-negative infections. The dorsal surface of the feet and the sole may also be affected.

CAT-SCRATCH DISEASE

Cat-scratch disease is a bacterial disorder caused by various subspecies of *Bartonella henselae* (formerly *Rochalimaea henselae*). *Afipia felis* may also induce the disease in a small number of patients.

Characteristically, the disease appears following contact with a cat. This contact (a scratch, bite or lick) is remembered in about 90% of patients. Cat-scratch disease is more frequent in children.

The upper limbs are the most common site of infection.

Clinical features

Cat-scratch disease is rare on the feet.

The primary lesion is polymorphic. It usually appears as an inflammatory papule or nodule which may ulcerate. Multiple primary lesions, often grouped together and of small size, may be observed, although these are very rare. Regional lymphadenopathy may be preceded by lymphangitis. The lymph nodes are enlarged, slightly tender and movable. These may also suppurate. Generalized lymphadenopathy or the involvement of lymph nodes in more than one region is rare.

Differential diagnosis

Because of the morphological nonspecificity of the primary lesion, the clinical diagnosis of cat-scratch disease is often difficult. A history of contact with a cat may be helpful. Histopathological examinations of both cutaneous lesions and, if necessary, lymph nodes, allow cat-scratch disease to be differentiated from bacterial lymphadenitis, atypical mycobacteriosis, sporotrichosis, toxoplasmosis, sarcoidosis, lymphomas etc.

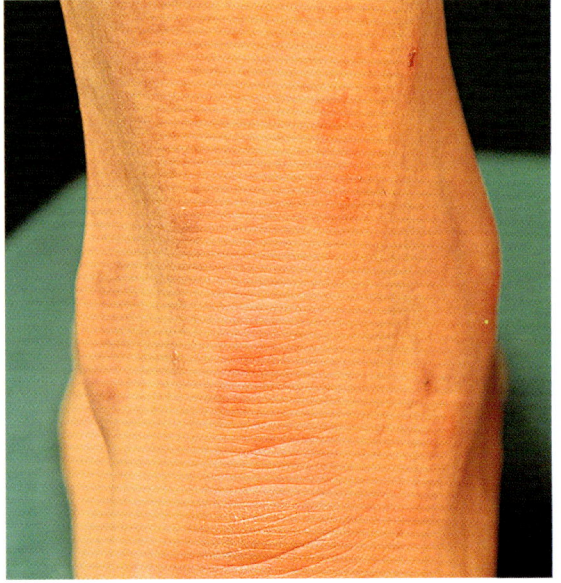

Figure 4.8
Cat-scratch disease. Multiple, erythematous, papules and nodules on the heel.

TUBERCULOSIS

Tuberculosis is a multisystemic disease caused by *Mycobacterium tuberculosis*. Cutaneous tuberculosis is the clinical outcome of the patient's immunological response to mycobacteria.

The classification of cutaneous tuberculosis depends essentially on the route of penetration of the mycobacteria into the skin. It is therefore possible to distinguish clinical varieties of cutaneous tuberculosis caused by the exogenous inoculation of mycobacteria (primary complex tuberculosis, verrucous tuberculosis and tuberculosis due to BCG vaccination) and clinical varieties due to the endogenous spread of mycobacteria (lupus vulgaris, scrofuloderma, orificial tuberculosis and miliary tuberculosis).

Clinical features

Of particular intertest is verrucous tuberculosis (tuberculosis verrucosa cutis). This is more frequent on the dorsal aspect of the fingers and hands, but the knees, ankles and dorsal aspect of the feet may also be affected, in particular in children and adolescents. The first lesion is a papule, nodule or plaque, highly variable in shape and size, reddish-violet in colour, parenchymatously-hard in consistency and asymptomatic. Seropurulent exudate and necrotic material may ooze. With time, the surface becomes irregular, verrucous and hyperkeratotic. Regional lymphadenopathy is not frequent but, when present, is nonsuppurative and asymptomatic. Long-standing infections may involve deep tissues (e.g. joints and bone). The development of squamous-cell carcinomas is also possible.

Differential diagnosis

Diagnosis of verrucous tuberculosis is essentially based on histopathological criteria. *Mycobacterium tuberculosis* may not be found, but can grow on culture. A skin test is positive. Polymerase chain reaction (PCR) is also positive in tissue specimens for *Mycobacterium tuberculosis* DNA. Other clinical varieties of cutaneous tuberculosis, chromoblastomycosis, hypertrophic lichen planus, pyoderma gangrenosum and squamous cell carcinoma are the most important diseases that enter into the differential diagnosis of verrucous tuberculosis.

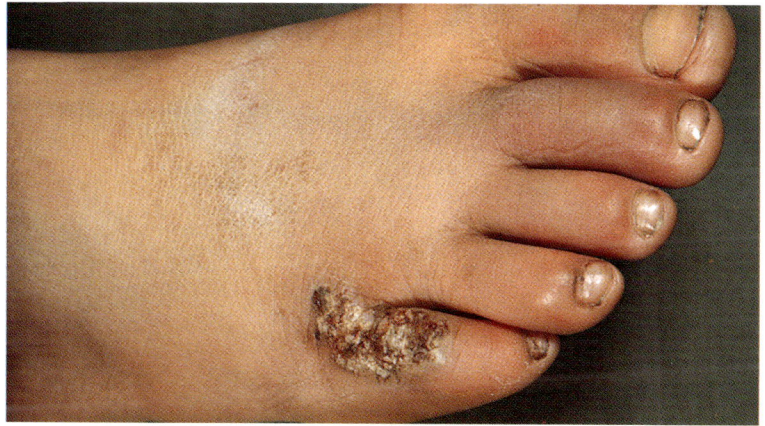

Figure 4.9
Verrucous tuberculosis. A verrucous-crusted lesion at the fifth toe.

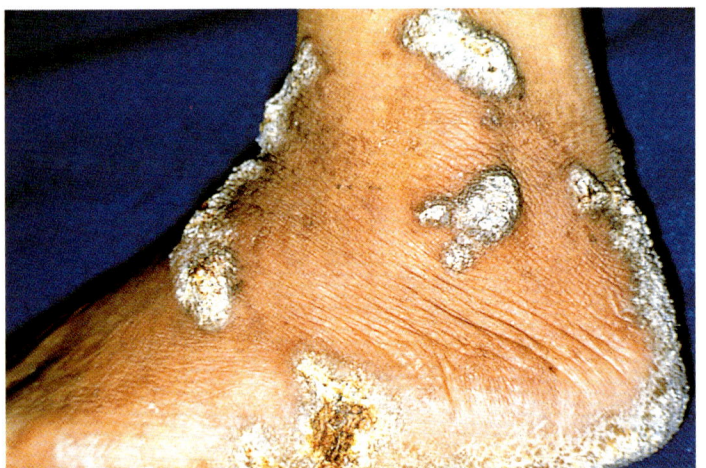

Figure 4.10
Verrucous tuberculosis. Multiple verrucous and hyperkeratotic lesions.

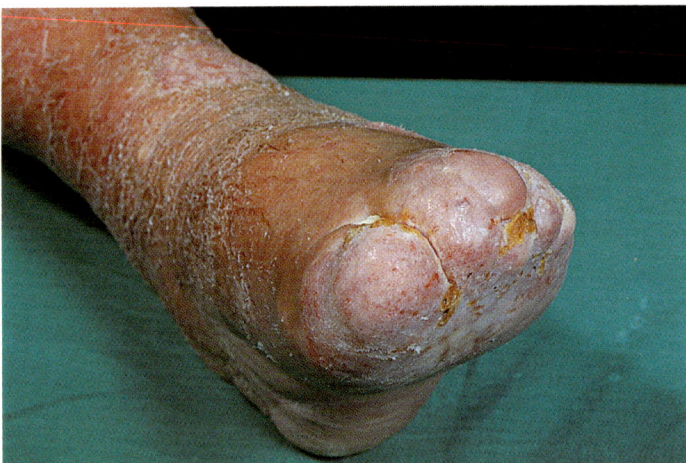

Figure 4.11
Verrucous tuberculosis. Disfigurement of the toes due to partial joint and bone destruction.

SYPHILIS

Syphilis is a sexually-transmitted disease caused by *Treponema pallidum*. It is characterized by three clinical stages (primary, secondary and tertiary syphilis). Furthermore, two other clinical varieties (congenital and latent (early and late) syphilis) must be considered.

The feet are typically involved in congenital and secondary syphilis.

Clinical features

Congenital syphilis is characterized by a mildly inflammatory, vesiculobullous eruption on the palms and soles. Subsequently, these lesions become moist erosions and eventually scales and crusts.

Secondary syphilis presents with an erythematous, papular, desquamative eruption on the palms and soles. The papules are round, pink, brown or copper-coloured, have a white collarette, are slightly firm, isolated or grouped together and asymptomatic.

Differential diagnosis

Secondary syphillis may present with polymorphic lesions (e.g. condylomata lata) involving the skin, hair and mucous membranes. Furthermore, numerous signs and symptoms may accompany the cutaneous eruption (conjunctivitis, pharyngitis, lymphadenopathy, hepatosplenomegaly, periostitis, meningitis, arrhythmias, fever, arthralgia, etc). Diagnosis of secondary syphilis is confirmed by dark field examination of exudate obtained from the moist lesions and by specific serology.

Other papulosquamous diseases that must be considered in differential diagnosis are mononucleosis, viral and drug-induced exanthemas, pityriasis rosea, guttate psoriasis and lichen planus.

Congenital syphilis must be distinguished from scabies.

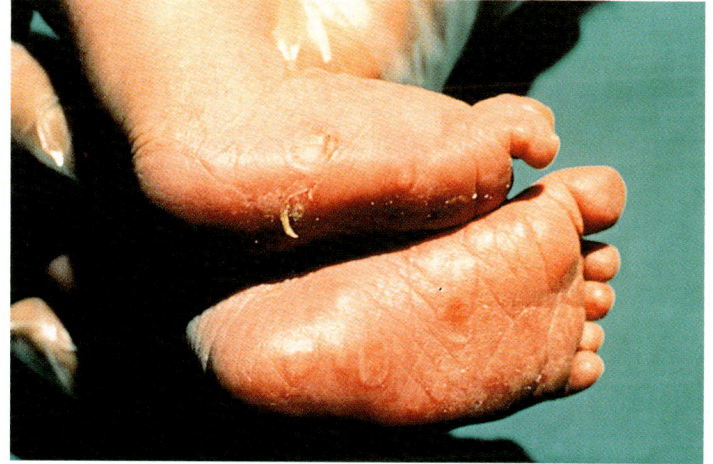

Figure 4.12

Congenital syphilis. Erosions are usually preceded by vesicles and bullae.

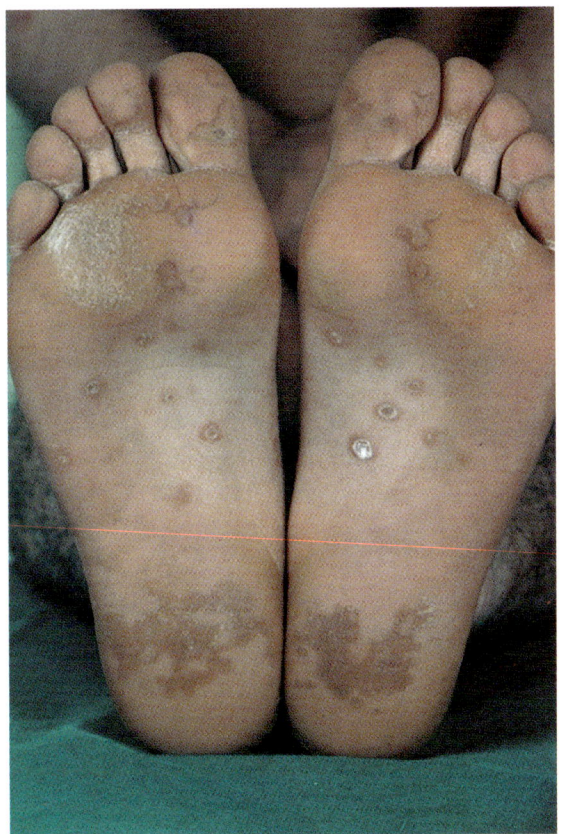 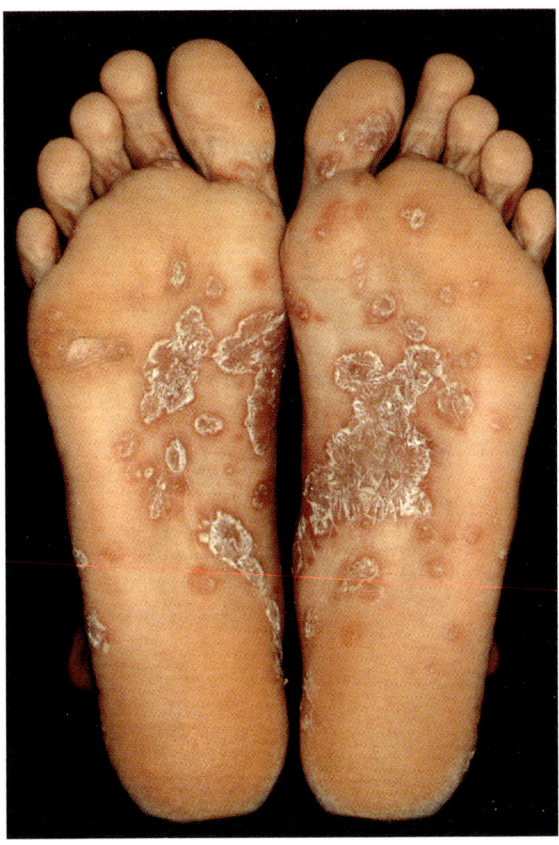

Figures 4.13 and 4.14

Secondary syphilis. Multiple, slightly inflammatory papules are circumscribed by a well-developed white collarette.

TINEA PEDIS

Tinea pedis (TP) is a superficial mycosis of the feet caused by various species of dermatophytes. *Trichophyton rubrum*, *T. mentagrophytes* and *Epidermophyton floccosum* are the most frequently involved species.

TP is more frequent in young males.

Sweating, poor hygiene, occlusive shoes and boots, and hot and humid weather represent the most important predisposing factors to the disease.

Clinical features

TP occurs exclusively on the feet. It is characterized by a macerative, erythematous and desquamative area initially located at third and/or fourth interdigital spaces.

Subsequently, this area undergoes erosion and fissuration. These manifestations are often accompanied by pruritus and burning. From the web spaces, the disease may spread as a vesiculobullous eruption to both the dorsal aspect of the feet and the soles. Chronic TP is characterized by erythematous, desquamative and hyperkeratotic lesions, which can involve the feet's entire skin surface.

Differential diagnosis

Clinical diagnosis should be confirmed by Wood's lamp, and by direct and cultural mycological examinations.

In allergic contact dermatitis and pompholyx, Wood's lamp and mycological examinations are negative.

Gram-negative infections of the feet, especially those caused by *Pseudomonas aeruginosa*, present with a characteristic greenish discharge accompanied by a bad smell. Gram's stain and bacteriological cultures confirm the diagnosis.

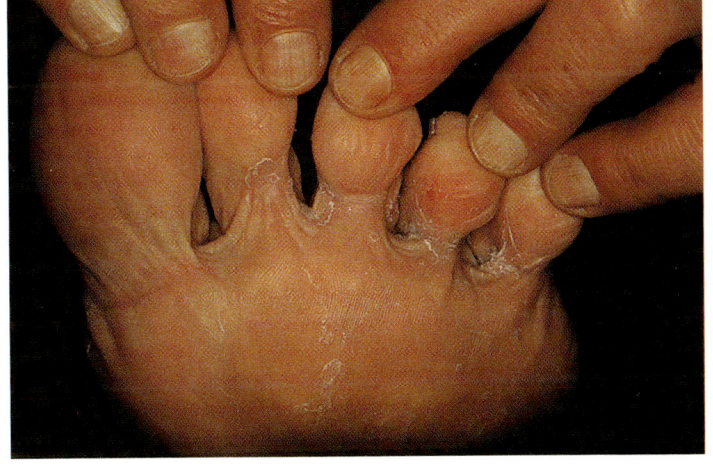

Figures 4.15 and 4.16

Tinea pedis. Development of erosions on macerative and desquamative areas at interdigital folds.

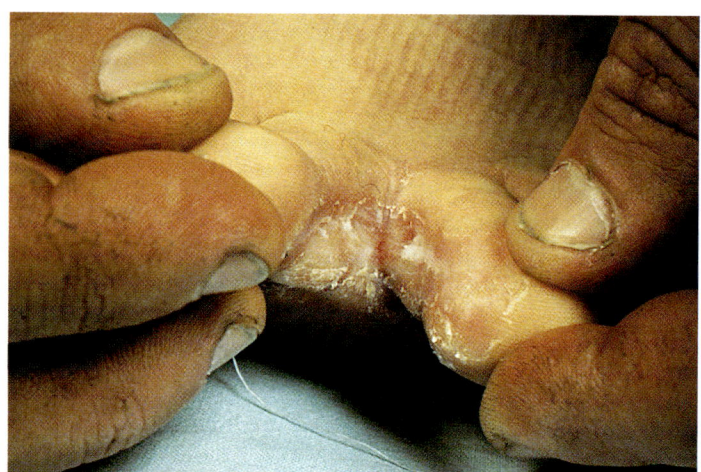

Figure 4.16
Tinea pedis.

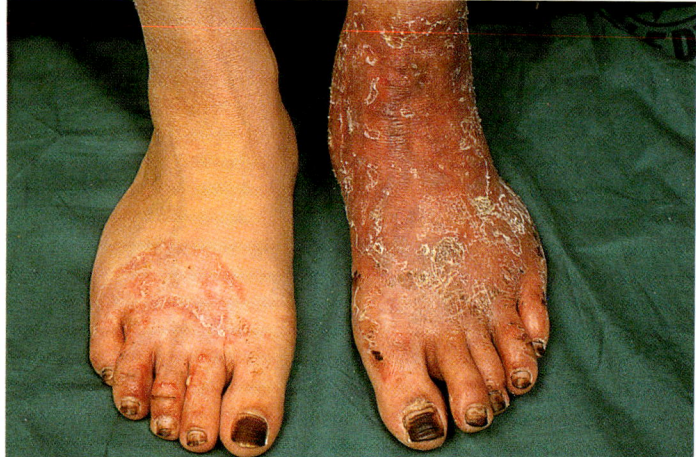

Figure 4.17
Tinea pedis. Chronic infections can involve the entire skin surface of the dorsum of the feet.

CANDIDIASIS

Candidiasis is mostly caused by *Candida albicans*, although other species of *Candida* are emerging.

Clinical features

Candidiasis is initially located in the interdigital spaces. From this site it can spread to the back of the feet and soles. The clinical picture is characterized by bright-red erythema, which undergoes erosion and fissure formation. A white, macerated collarette is present at the periphery of the lesions. Pruritus and pain are characteristic.

Often associated with interdigital candidiasis is paronychia. This develops initially on one toe only. Periungual tissues appear erythematous and oedematous. Small pockets of pus are present. Upon applying pressure, a creamy, white-yellow exudate may be expressed. Pain may be severe. The infection usually extends to the nail-plate. Proximal and lateral portions of the nail-plate present with a yellow-green or yellow-brown pigmentation. The nail becomes thickened and its surface becomes irregular.

Differential diagnosis

Direct and cultural examinations allow candidiasis to be distinguished from tinea pedis, bacterial intertrigo, psoriasis, allergic contact dermatitis and pompholyx.

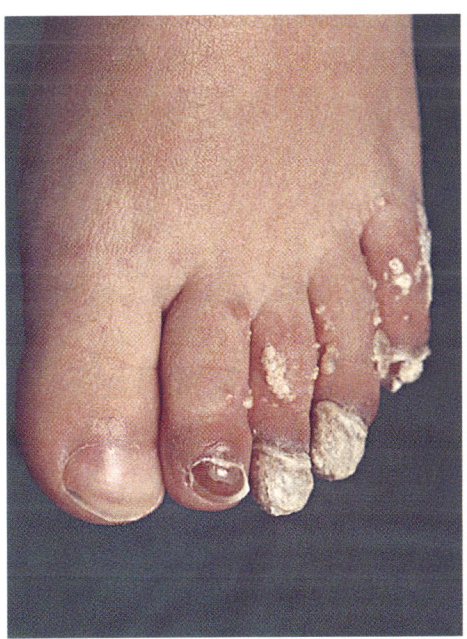

Figure 4.18
Paronychia. Periungual tissue appears erythematous and oedematous.

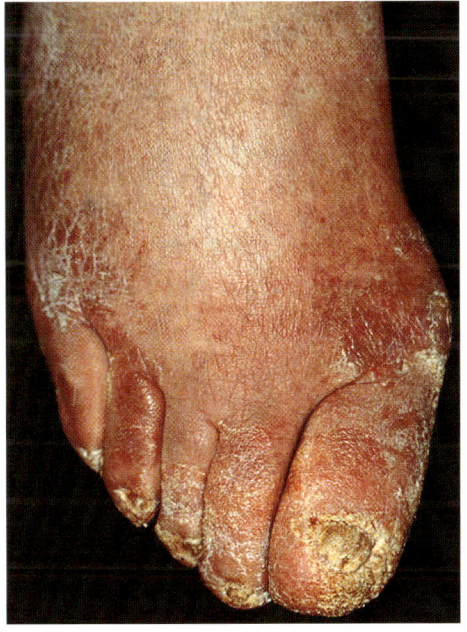

Figure 4.19
Paronychia. Nail-plates appear discoloured and thickened.

SPOROTRICHOSIS

Sporotrichosis is a disease caused by *Sporothrix schenckii*, a fungus that lives as a saprophyte in the soil and on numerous plants. The upper limbs (the dorsal aspect of the fingers and hand, wrist and forearm) are the most frequent sites of infection.

The fungus penetrates the skin through minor traumas caused by thorns or wooden splinters. Sporotrichosis usually occurs in farmers and gardeners. It may therefore be considered a work-related disease.

Clinical features

Sporotrichosis on the feet is rare. At the site of inoculation, a papule, nodule or plaque appears. This is mildly inflammatory, parenchymatous-hard in consistency and asymptomatic. With time, the primary lesion enlarges and then ulcerates. A few weeks later similar, although deeper and sometimes ulcerated, nodules develop along the lymphatics (sporotrichoid lymphangitis). Finally, a regional suppurative lymphadenitis occurs. Fistulae formation is not uncommon.

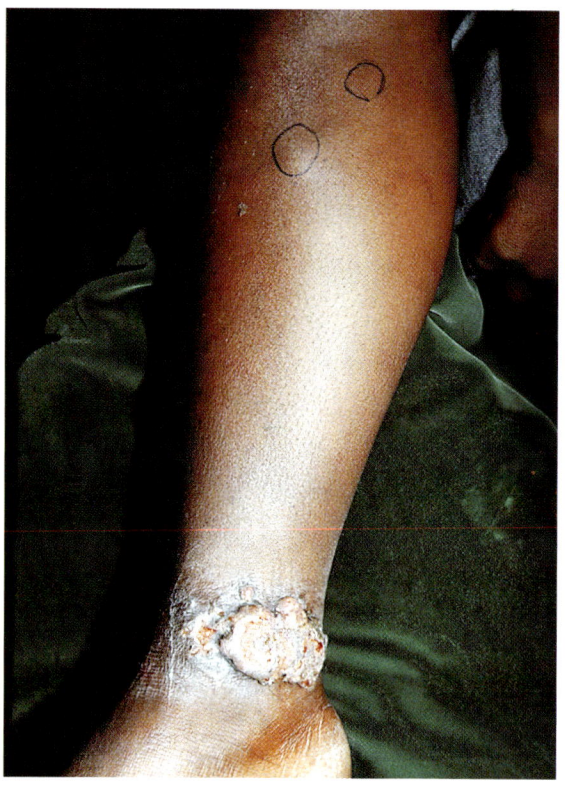

Figure 4.20
Sporotrichosis. A vegetating mass at the ankle.

Differential diagnosis

The primary lesion must be distinguished from cutaneous tuberculosis, atypical mycobacteriosis, cat-scratch disease and cutaneous leishmaniasis. A biopsy for histopathological examination and cultures for bacteria, fungi and protozoa are always necessary.

'Sporotrichoid' atypical mycobacteriosis has to be taken into consideration in the differential diagnosis of lymphangitic sporotrichosis.

CHROMOBLASTOMYCOSIS

Chromoblastomycosis (or chromomycosis) is a mycosis caused by fungi belonging to various families: *Phialophora* sp., *Fonsecaea* sp. and *Chladosporium* sp. are the fungi most frequently responsible for the disease.

Transmission of chromoblastomycosis is a consequence of the skin coming into contact with moist soil, wood or leaves. Recurrent, post-traumatic lesions are a predisposing factor. The disease is endemic in moist areas of Central and South America, where it is considered an occupational disease. Chromoblastomycosis in fact almost exclusively affects farmers, woods-men and foresters.

Adult males are the people most commonly affected.

Clinical features

The legs and feet are, by far, the most frequent sites affected by chromoblastomycosis. Cutaneous lesions are polymorphic. Noninflammatory papules, nodules and plaques, often with a rugged verrucous surface, develop on the legs and dorsal aspect of the feet. These enlarge and undergo ulceration, with secondary bacterial superinfection. Scarring, hyper- and/or hypopigmented macules and elephantiasis as a result of underlying oedema and lymphoedema represent the final outcome of the disease.

Onychodystrophies are also frequent.

All cutaneous lesions may be asymptomatic.

Squamous cell carcinomas can develop on chronic lesions.

Differential diagnosis

The diagnosis of chromoblastomycosis is based on clinical, histopathological and mycological criteria. Numerous other infectious diseases may enter into differential diagnosis with chromoblastomycosis (e.g. verrucous tuberculosis, leprosy, botryomycosis, sporotrichosis, lobomycosis, mycetomas, etc).

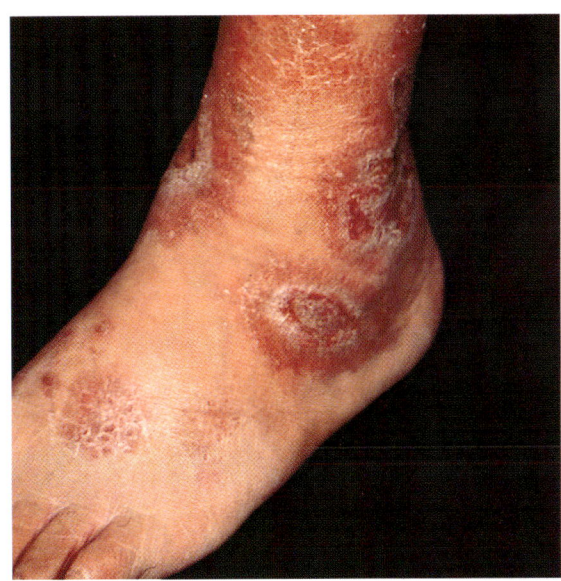

Figure 4.21
Chromoblastomycosis. Multiple nodules and plaques.

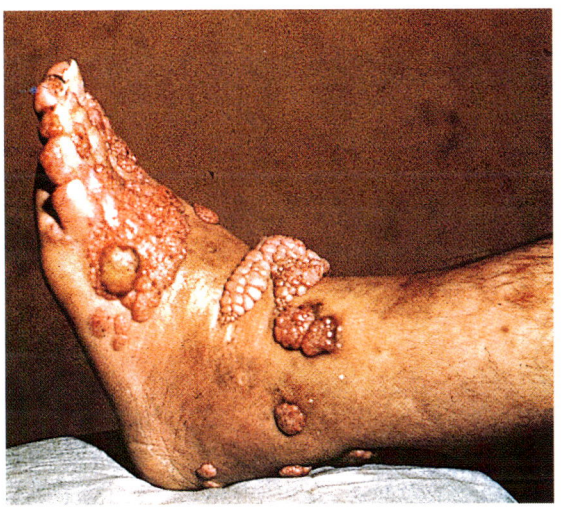

Figure 4.22
Chromoblastomycosis. Vegetating and verrucous nodules on an oedematous and lymphoedematous base.

MYCETOMAS

Mycetomas are cutaneous, subcutaneous and deep diseases caused by numerous micro-organisms that produce granules. According to the aetiological agent involved, mycetomas may be classified into actinomycotic mycetomas, caused by actinomycetes (among others: *Actinusmadurae* sp., *Nocardia* sp. and *Streptomyces* sp.), and eumycotic mycetomas, caused by fungi (among others: *Aspergillus* sp., *Fusarium* sp., *Madurella* sp. and *Phialophora* sp.). Botryomocoses are caused by true bacteria and therefore are not considered to belong to the mycetomas group.

Mycetomas are common in tropical and subtropical countries, where they particularly infect adult agricultural workers who walk barefoot. These diseases are, in fact, caused by the transcutaneous inoculation of micro-organisms following thorn pricks or wooden splinters. The feet, therefore, represent the most common site of infection. The legs and hands may also be affected.

Clinical features

The primary lesions may be located on the back of the foot or the sole, and is characterized by a papule, nodule or plaque that enlarges and then ulcerates. These ulcers exude a pus that contains granules called 'grains'. These are small masses of micro-organism colonies of different colours (white, yellow, red, brown, black according to the aetiological agent). These manifestations are accompanied by oedema, lymphoedema and bacterial superinfections. Regional lymphadenopathy and fever may also be present. In patients with long-standing disease, the infection can spread to deep tissues (fascia, muscle and bone).

Differential diagnosis

Diagnosis of mycetoma is based on mycology (direct examination of pus and grains, and cultures for *Actinomycetales* and fungi) and histopathological examination. Instrumental investigations (echography, X-ray) are also helpful.

Mycetomas enter into the differential diagnosis of several tropical and subtropical infectious diseases (verrucous tuberculosis, leprosy, deep mycoses and leishmaniasis). Pyoderma gangrenosum should also be considered in differential diagnosis.

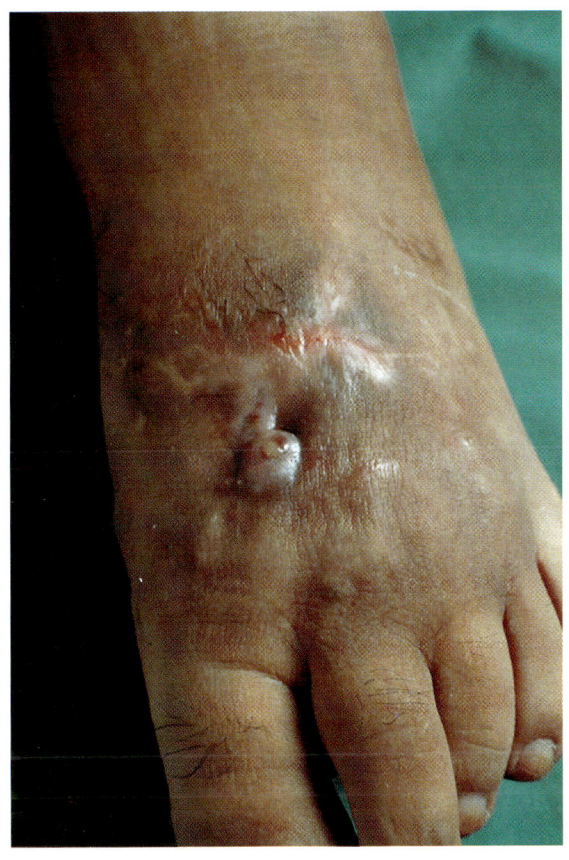

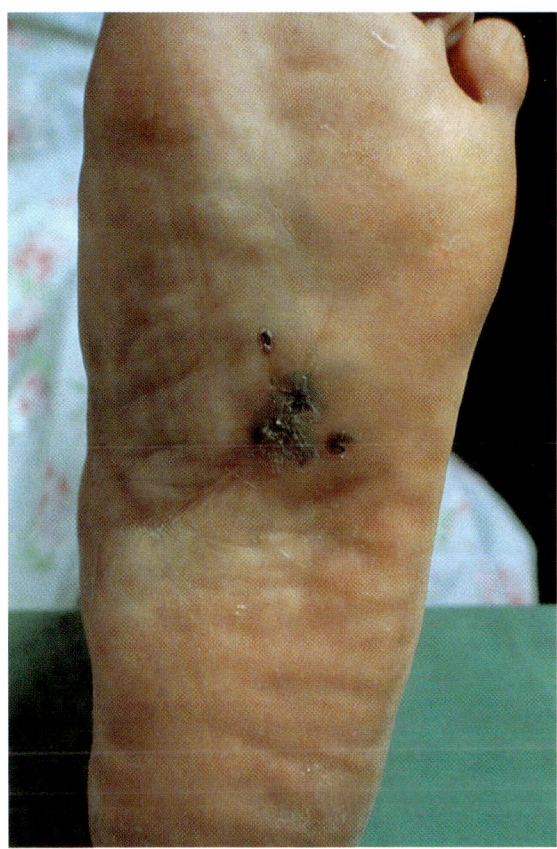

Figure 4.23
Eumycotic mycetoma. An ulcerated plaque draining a purulent exudate containing grains.

Figure 4.24
Eumycotic mycetoma. A plaque on the sole: large black grains may be observed.

PRIMARY HERPES SIMPLEX

The first contact of the skin and/or mucous membranes with herpes simplex virus (HSV) may be expressed as an asymptomatic infection or as clinical manifestations (primary herpes simplex – PHS). The oral cavity, in particular the gums (herpetic gingivostomatitis) and the eyes, particularly the conjunctiva (herpetic keratoconjunctivitis) are the most frequent sites for PHS infection. In most cases, PHS is characterized by a mild clinical picture. Children are mainly affected.

Clinical features

PHS is extremely rare on the feet. Following a transitory phase characterized by erythema and oedema, the first vesicles appear. They are round, surrounded by an erythematous halo and grouped together. Subsequently, they may become erosions or pustules and, later, crusts. All lesions heal in 2–4 weeks, leaving a transitory brown hyperpigmentation. Scarring is very rare. Pain and burning are severe. Regional lymphadenopathy, general malaise, fever, headache, arthralgia and myalgia are quite frequent.

Differential diagnosis

Hand-foot-and-mouth disease, herpangina, Kawasaki's disease, aphthous stomatitis, fixed-drug eruption and erythema multiforme must be considered in the differential diagnosis of PHS of the oral cavity. Impetigo can mimic PHS on the feet.

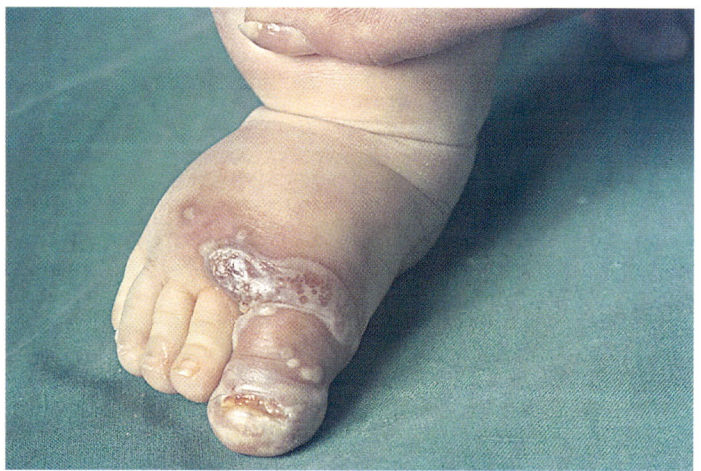

Figure 4.25
Primary herpes simplex. Grouped vesicles and pustules on an erythematous-oedematous base.

WARTS

Warts are infections caused by various types of human papilloma virus (HPV). They are very common in children and young adults. The face, the dorsal surfaces of the fingers and hands, and the soles are the most frequent sites of infection.

Plantar warts are usually caused by HPV types 1, 2 and 4.

Clinical features

Plantar warts may be either single or multiple, isolated or confluent. They appear as round, flattened papules and/or plaques, of variable size, whitish or grey in colour, with a rough surface. Removal (by means of a scalpel or keratolytic products) of the hyperkeratotic surface will reveal tiny, reddish-brown dots. Plantar warts are often intensely painful, both spontaneously and under pressure.

Differential diagnosis

Corns develop on the pressure areas of the sole. Dots are not visible following removal of the hyperkeratotic surface.

Tungiasis affects only those people who have come from areas where this infestation is endemic.

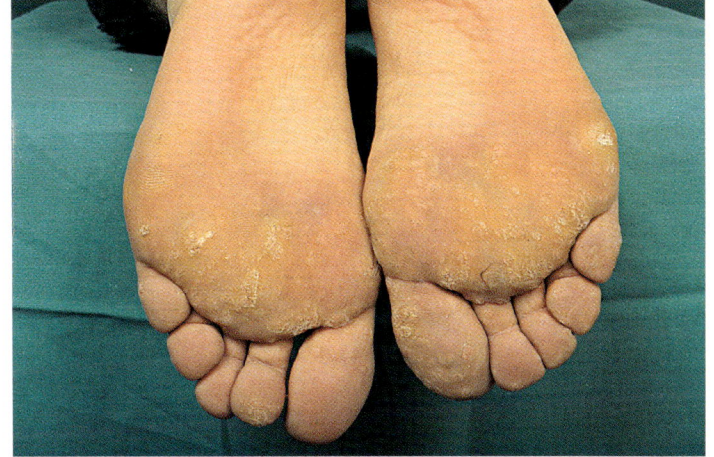

Figure 4.26
Plantar warts. Multiple hyperkeratotic plaques on the sole.

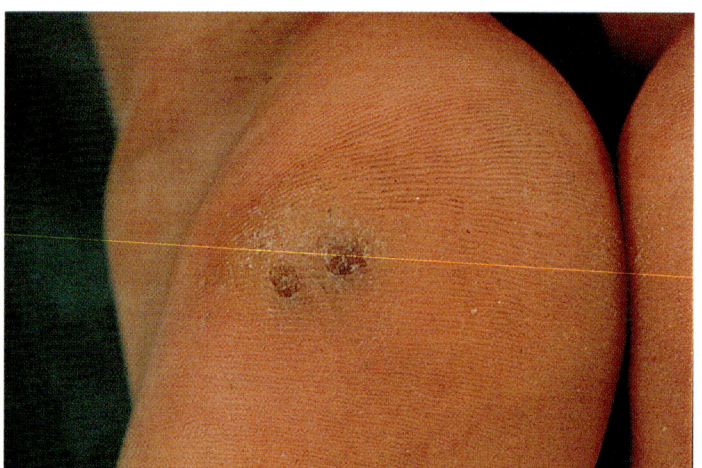

Figure 4.27
Plantar warts. Two greyish-black lesions on the heel.

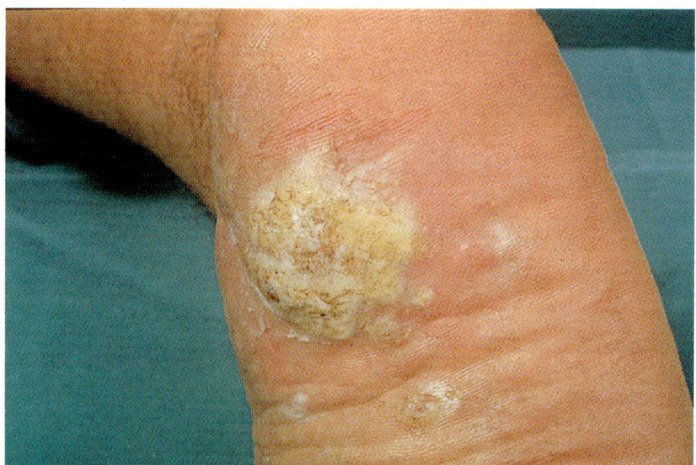

Figure 4.28
Plantar warts. Giant plantar wart in an immunocompromised patient.

HAND-FOOT-AND-MOUTH DISEASE

Hand-foot-and-mouth disease (HFMD) is caused by enteroviruses belonging to Coxsackie groups A and B. It almost exclusively occurs in children of preschool age. The disease manifests itself in seasonal (mainly summer) epidemics, in which serotype A16 is the virus most frequently involved. The disease is characterized by the sudden appearance of vesicles in the oral cavity (lips, tongue, cheeks, hard and soft palate, pharynx) and on the hands and feet – hence the name 'hand-foot-and-mouth disease'. The disease may be accompanied by malaise, low-grade fever and a mild burning sensation in the oral cavity.

Clinical features

The vesicles are mainly located on the heels and on the flexural surface of the fingers. They are round or, more frequently, oval, a few millimetres in size and surrounded by an erythematous halo. The content is serous and later purulent.

Differential diagnosis

Aphthous stomatitis is rare in children. It is characterized by painful ulcers that have a yellowish base and a marked erythematous halo. These lesions are larger and more painful than those of HFMD.

Herpes simplex is characterized by grouped vesicles which become postules and then erosions and crusts. Oral cavity involvement occurs almost exclusively in primary herpes simplex infection.

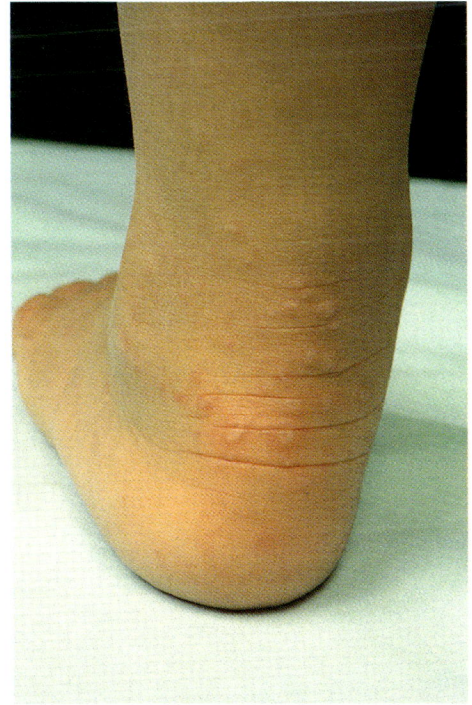

Figure 4.29
Hand-foot-and-mouth disease. Papulovesicular lesions, circumscribed by an erythematous halo, on the heel.

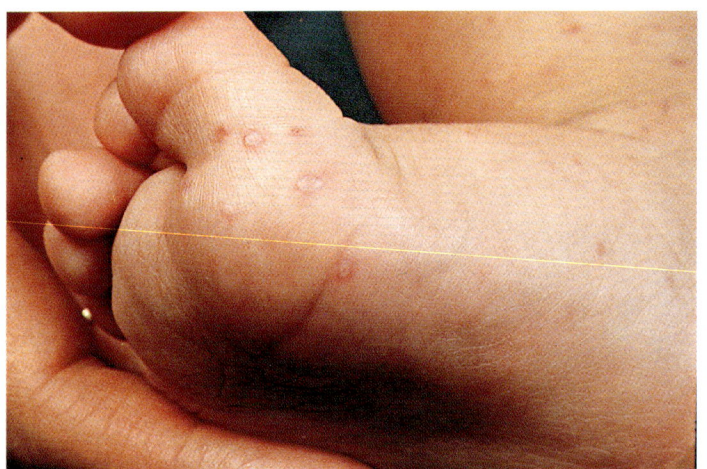

Figures 4.30 and 4.31
Hand-foot-and-mouth disease.
Round and oval lesions at the first
toe.

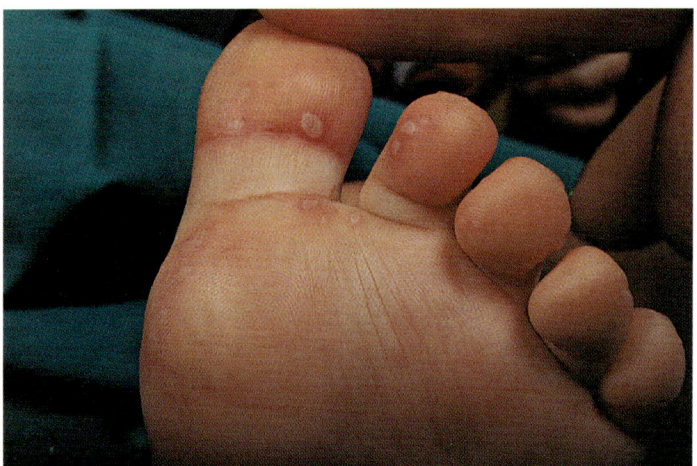

Figure 4.31
Hand-foot-and-mouth disease.

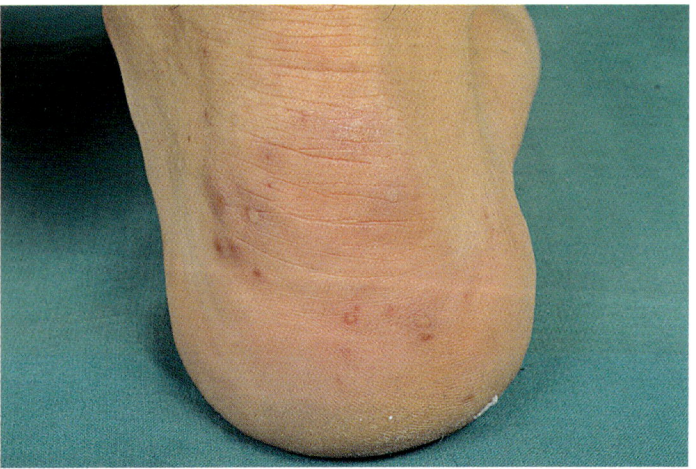

Figure 4.32
Hand-foot-and-mouth disease.
Healing lesions on the heel in an
adult patient.

PAPULAR-PURPURIC 'GLOVES AND SOCKS' SYNDROME

Papular-purpuric 'gloves and socks' syndrome (PPGSS) is caused by a variety of viruses (Coxsackie B 6, cytomegalovirus and measles virus), although human parvovirus B 19 is the virus most frequently encountered. PPGSS almost exclusively affects young Caucasian adults of both sexes during the spring.

Clinical features

Cutaneous manifestations are typical. Initially, oedema and erythema occur, symmetrically located on the hands and feet, in a glove-and-sock distribution. Subsequently, at the same sites, erythematouspapular, purpuric lesions appear. These are of a few millimetres in diameter and are isolated or confluent. They may be asymptomatic, pruritic or mildly painful. Nonspecific oral lesions may be present. Systemic symptoms (asthenia, headache, anorexia and arthralgia) and signs (fever and lymphadenopathy) are rare and mild in intensity.

Differential diagnosis

Erythema multiforme is characterized by the presence of target-like lesions. Oral manifestations are common.

Hand-foot-and-mouth disease presents with typical, oval, vesicular lesions in the oral cavity, hands and feet.

Childhood papular acrodermatitis (Gianotti–Crosti syndrome) may be associated with hepatitis B virus infection; its characteristic lesion is a papule.

PPGSS also enters into differential diagnosis with Rocky Mountain spotted fever (only in the USA) and Kawasaki's disease (very rare in adults).

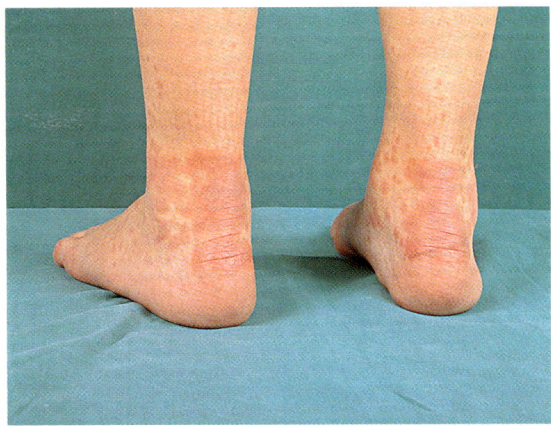

Figure 4.33
Papular-purpuric 'gloves and socks' syndrome. Oedema and erythema, symmetrically localized on the feet in a child.

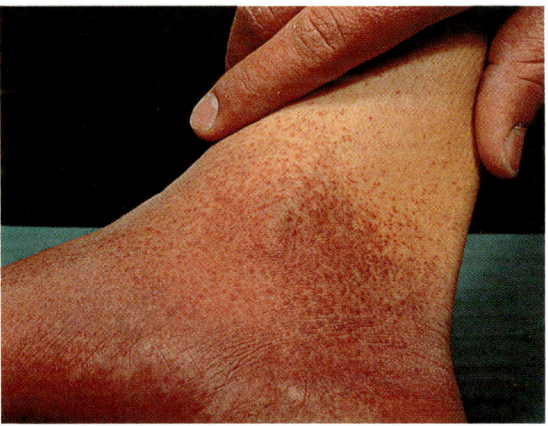

Figure 4.34
Papular-purpuric 'gloves and socks' syndrome. Typical purpuric papules arranged according to a sock distribution.

CUTANEOUS LARVA MIGRANS

Cutaneous larva migrans (CLM) is an infestation that results because of the penetration and migration into the skin of nematode larvae. *Ancylostoma braziliense* and *A. caninum* are the most frequent species.

The feet, ankles and buttocks are the most common sites of infestation.

Clinical features

CLM is characterized clinically by slightly raised tracks. These are erythematous, linear or more often, serpiginous, ramified and intertwined. They are of variable length (often many centimetres) and width (usually 2–4 mm). Papules (mainly at the site of penetration of the larvae), vesicles and bullae (especially along the tracks) may be observed.

Pruritus is always present and often severe.

Differential diagnosis

Larva currens, caused by *Strongyloides stercoralis* occurs mainly on the anal and perianal region, buttocks, inguinal folds and thighs. Often associated with this are an urticarial rash or frank urticaria, and a papular, purpuric eruption. Pruritus is diffuse and sometimes intolerable.

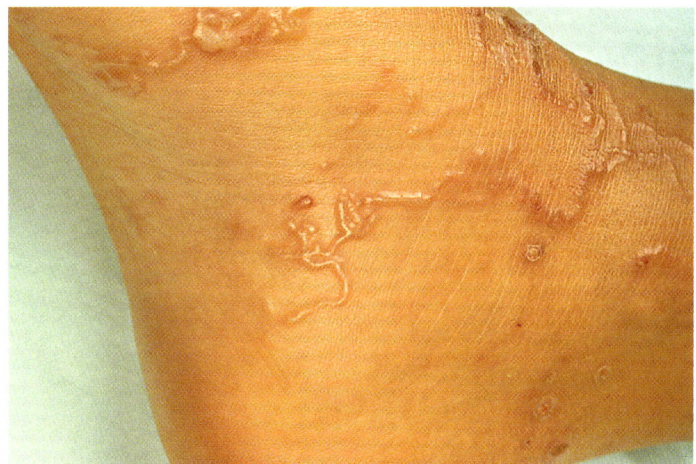

Figures 4.35 and 4.36
Cutaneous larva migrans.
Serpiginous and intertwined tracks.

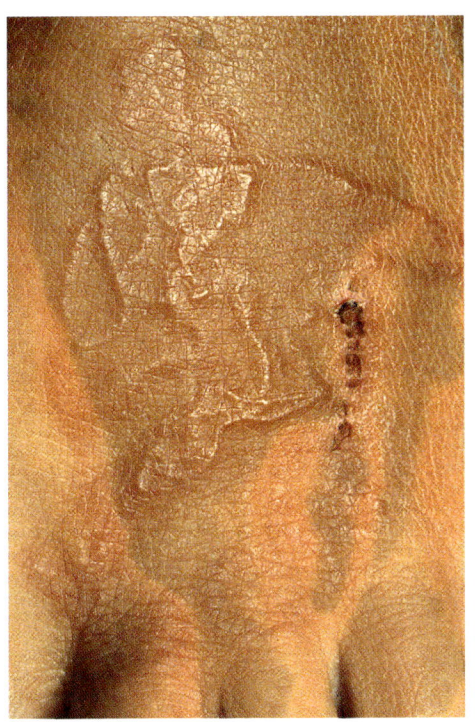

Figure 4.36
Cutaneous larva migrans.

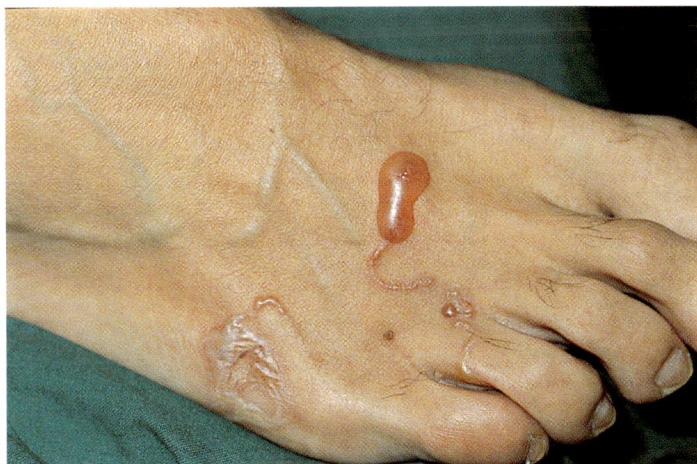

Figure 4.37
Cutaneous larva migrans. A
bullous lesion along a track.

FILARIASIS

Under the term filariasis, at least three diseases are included, according to the nematode that is responsible for the disease. These nematodes are *Wuchereria bancrofti*, *Brugia malayi* and *B. timori*.

Filariasis caused by *Wuchereria bancrofti* is by far the most common clinical variety, occuring in more than 90 million patients.

The disease is transmitted by mosquitoes belonging to the genera *Aedes*, *Anopheles*, *Culex* and *Mansonia*.

Clinical manifestations of filariasis are the result of mechanical factors (subocclusion and occlusion of the lymphatics caused by adult nematodes) as well as toxic and allergic phenomena (sensitization of the patient against metabolic products that are released by adult nematodes during their moults).

Clinical features

The lower limbs are mostly affected by filariasis. Swelling and inflammatory lymphoedema, acute lymphangitis and acute nonsuppurative lymphadenitis represent the first manifestations of the disease. With time, all these manifestations become chronic and recurrent. The final outcome is represented by elphantiasis, generally involving both lower limbs from the groin down to the feet. The skin appears hypertrophic, xerotic, verrucous and hard in consistency. Spontaneous and post-traumatic ulcerations followed by bacterial superinfections are common.

Differential diagnosis

Filariasis must be differentiated from all those diseases that cause elephantiasis (e.g. other infestations caused by nematodes, lymphangitis, lymphadenitis, erysipelas (elephantiasis vostra streptogenes), lymph node metastases from malignant tumours, venous stasis and other diseases of vessels.

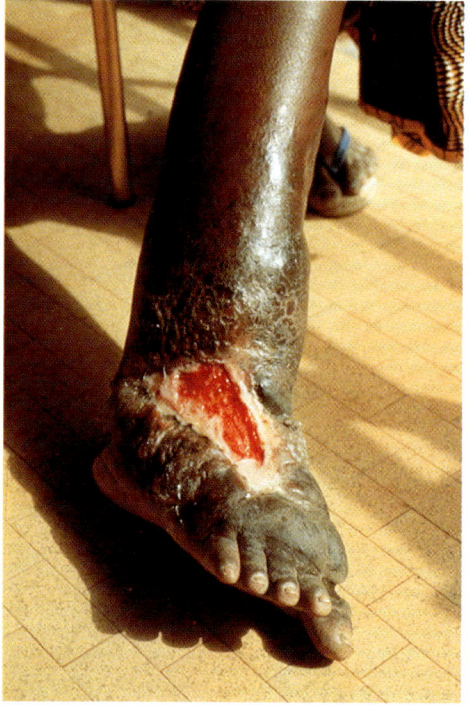

Figure 4.38

Filariasis. Elephantiasis with a wide and deep ulcer caused by *Wuchereria bancrofti*.

FLEA INFESTATIONS

Flea infestations are mainly caused by *Pulex irritans*.

Infestation is more frequent in tropical and subtropical climates and, in temperate climates, during the summer.

The legs, ankles and feet are the sites most characteristically affected. This is due to the fact that fleas lack wings but they do have a well-developed third pair of legs. This allows fleas to perform bounds up to 30 cm.

Clinical features

Flea bites present with erythematous wheals or papules. These are round, red in colour, with a tiny central ulcer corresponding to the sting site.

The lesions are isolated or grouped randomly. The development of vesicles and/or bullae is not common, but erythematous, papular, purpuric lesions frequently appear, especially on the legs, ankles and feet of adults. Flea infestations are always very pruritic. Common findings are linear excoriations as a result of scratching and secondary bacterial superinfections.

Differential diagnosis

Bedbug stings present with groups of two or three erythematous wheals or papules, with a small central ulcer, arranged in a row (breakfast, lunch and dinner or three-meal disease).

Other insects that can provoke skin reactions clinically similar to those caused by fleas are mosquitoes and horseflies.

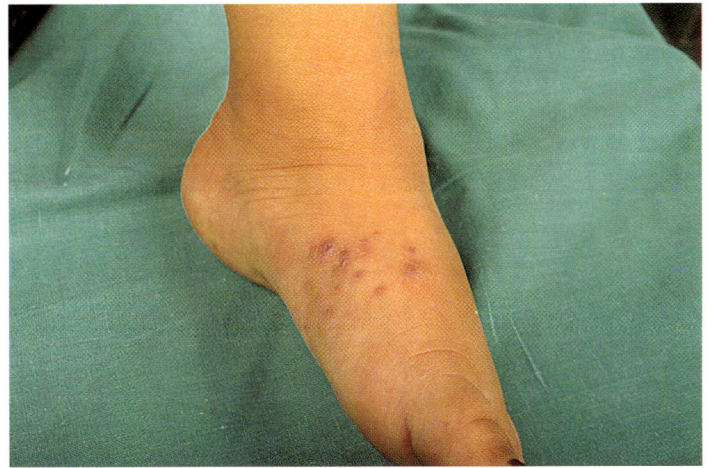

Figure 4.39
Flea infestation. A group of papulovesicular lesions on the dorsal aspect of the foot.

TUNGIASIS

Tungiasis is an infestation of the skin and nail apparatus caused by the female flea of *Tunga penetrans*. The most common sites of infestation are the sub- and periungual folds of the toes, sole, interdigital spaces and heels. Other sites of infestation are the legs, knees, thighs and hands.

Clinical features

The infestation is characterized clinically by a papular or nodular lesion. This is round, a few millimetres in diameter, white, yellowish, grey or black in colour, with a central brown-black tiny opening corresponding to the posterior portion of the flea. By enlarging this opening and by exerting pressure at the sides, it is possible to remove fragments of the inset, eggs and necrotic material. Its consistency is parenchymatous-hard. The lesion may also be erythematous, pustular, ulcerative or crusted. Bacterial superinfection is not uncommon. Pain is frequent and often severe. Walking may be markedly limited.

Differential diagnosis

Patients with tungiasis have always returned from a trip to Central and South America, sub-Saharan Africa or central Asia.

Warts occur mainly on the sole (plantar warts). These may be either single or multiple and appear clinically as skin-coloured papules and/or plaques, with a rough surface and tiny, reddish-brown dots. These dots are often only visible by removing (by means of a scalpel or keratic products) the hyperkeratotic surface. Plantar warts are also tender. Biopsy for histopathological examination is sometimes necessary.

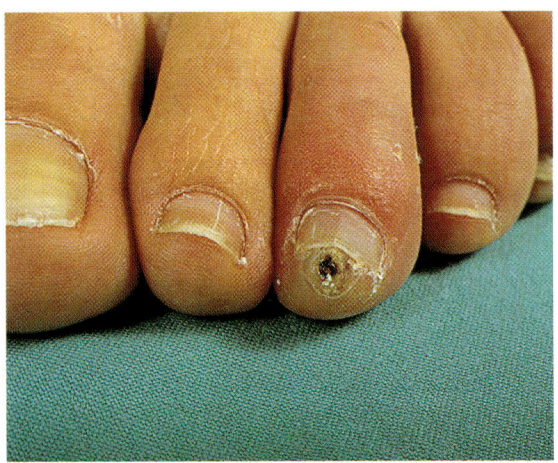

Figure 4.40
Tungiasis. A central brown-black opening circumscribed by a hyperkeratotic ring.

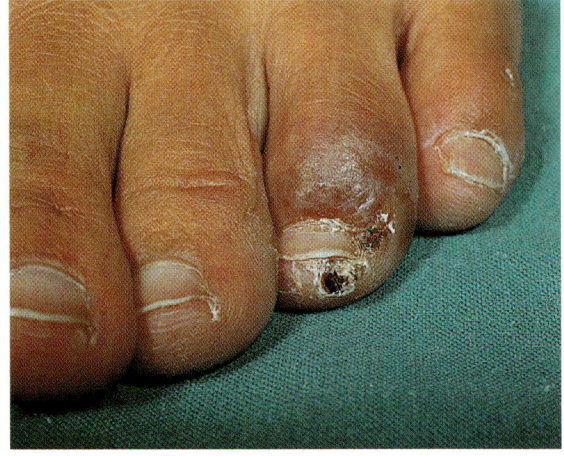

Figure 4.41
Tungiasis. The swelling suggests a bacterial superinfection.

SCABIES

Scabies is an infestation caused by the female of the mite *Sarcoptes scabiei* var. *hominis.* This is a very common pruritic disease with a worldwide distribution.

Clinical features

In adults, scabies can sometimes occur on the back of the feet with the usual clinical manifestations (burrows, papular and vesicular lesions, excoriations with a linear arrangement due to scratching and pustular lesions caused by bacterial superinfections). In infants, the involvement of the feet, in particular the soles, is very characteristic. In infants scabies can also present with a variety of clinical lesions, in particular papules and vesicles but also bullae, pustules, erosions, scaling and crusts.

Norwegian scabies (crusted scabies) is characterized by verrucous and crusted lesions located, among other sites, on the feet. Pruritus may be mild or absent.

Differential diagnosis

Clinical diagnosis of scabies must be confirmed by microscopic evidence of mites or their eggs or faeces. However, in a small number of patients, microscopic examinations are sometimes negative, possibly because of the very low number of parasites involved. Abundance of mites is characteristic of immunocompromised patients.

The diseases that have to be considered in the differential diagnosis of scabies include pediculosis, dermatitis herpetiformis and papular urticaria. Norwegian scabies must be differentiated from atopic dermatitis, psoriasis, seborrhoeic dermatitis and Langerhans' cell histiocytosis.

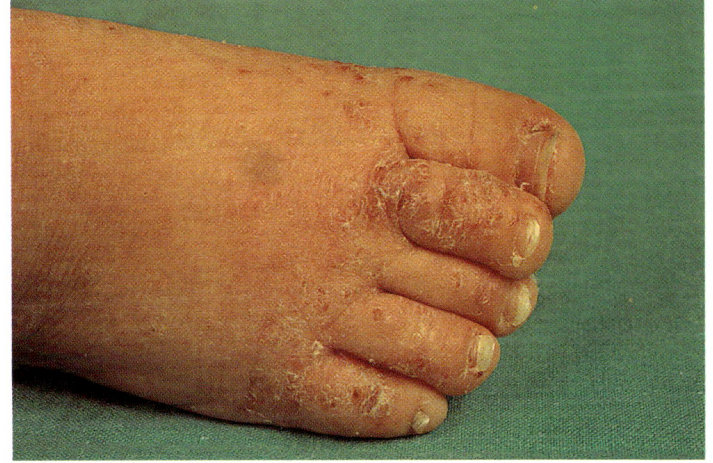

Figure 4.42
Scabies. The presence of crusts is due to scratching.

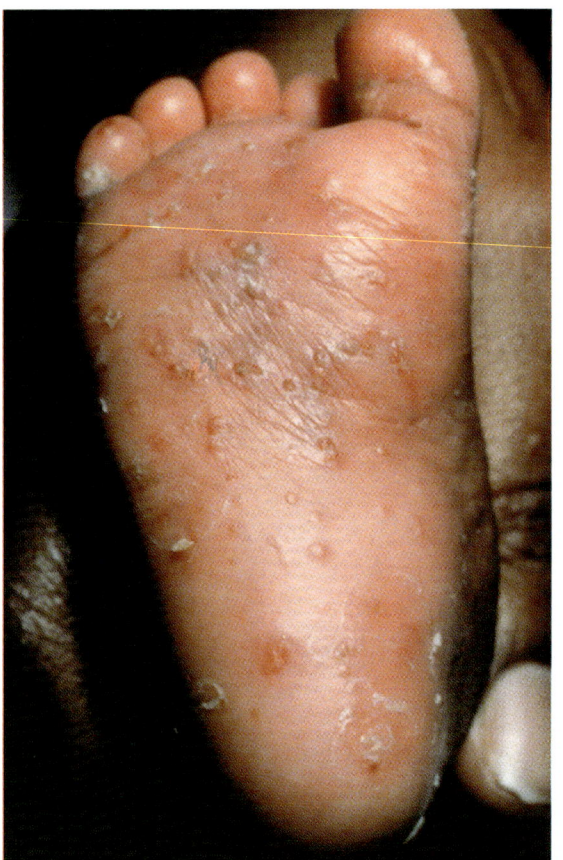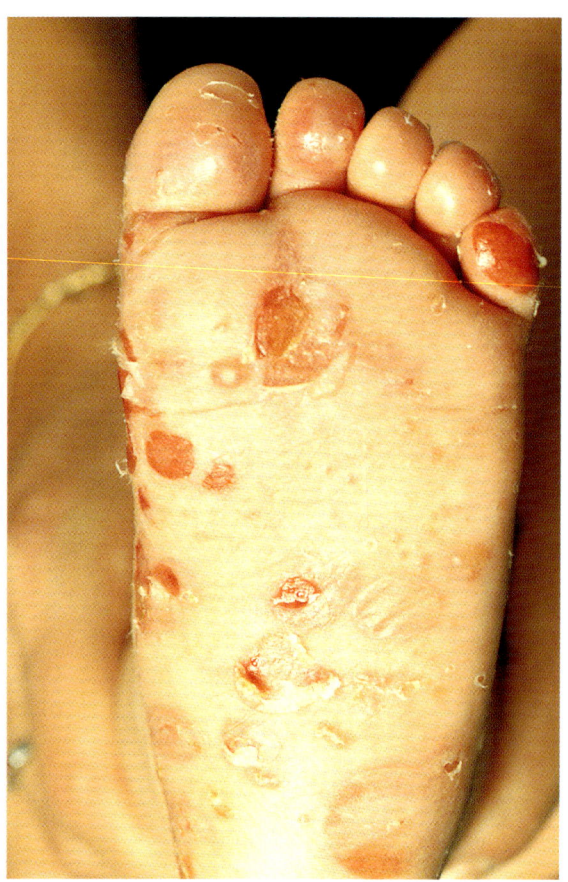

Figure 4.43 and 4.44
Scabies. Vesicular and bullous lesions are characteristically localized on the soles.

JELLYFISH INFESTATIONS

Cutaneous manifestations as a result of contact with the tentacles of jellyfish are becoming more and more frequent. All skin surface may be affected, perhaps with the exception of the areas of the body covered by the bathing suit.

Systemic involvement is possible.

Clinical features

The arrangement of the lesions reflects the contact made with the jellyfish tentacles: these may be linear, tuft-like or have a lash-like appearance. The morphology of the lesions, although nonspecific, is characteristic. The rash varies in composition from erythematous and urticarial lesions to vesicular, bullous, erosive and ulcerative, necrotic lesions. More or less severe burning and pain are always present. A transitory postinflammatory hyperpigmentation is common but scarring is rare.

Differential diagnosis

The diagnosis of jellyfish-induced dermatitis is almost always made by the patient him or herself, who at first complains of an acute sensation of burning and/or pain and then notices the appearance of inflammatory lesions at the sites of contact.

Other marine animals belonging to the phylum coelenterates, such as anemones and corals, have to be considered as possible aetiological agents in these types of rash.

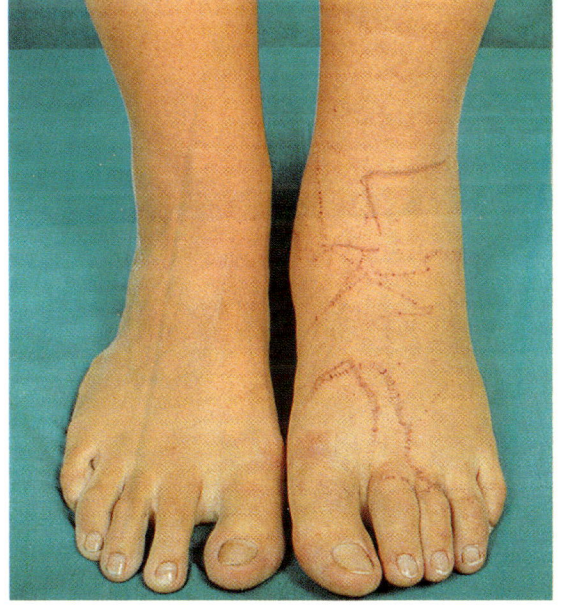

Figure 4.45
Jellyfish infestations. Typical linear or lash-like arrangement of the lesions.

5 Miscellaneous disorders

PHYSIOLOGICAL SCALING OF THE NEWBORN
DIGITAL ABNORMALITIES
PRIMARY CUTANEOUS LOCALIZED AMYLOIDOSIS
GOUT
LIPOATROPHY
PIEZOGENIC PEDAL PAPULES
PARANEOPLASTIC ACROKERATOSIS
LIVEDO RETICULARIS
VENOUS ULCERS
ATHEROSCLEROTIC ISCHAEMIC LESIONS
DIABETIC FOOT
LYMPHOEDEMA
HYPERTENSIVE ULCERS
ARTERIOVENOUS FISTULA
ARTERIAL EMBOLIC ISCHAEMIC LESIONS
CHRONIC PERNIOSIS
HENNA

PHYSIOLOGICAL SCALING OF THE NEWBORN

Physiological scaling of the newborn is the most common skin finding of the neonatal period, occurring in about 75% of normal neonates. Desquamation is usually localized to the ankles, feet and hands and it is characterized by noninflammatory, white, thin, fine scales. It tends to be more severe in postmature infants. Physiological scaling resolves within a few days and up to 2 weeks after birth.

Differential diagnosis

Congenital ichthyoses may be differentiated by family history, the persistence of scaling beyond the first few weeks, the scales' appearance and their different distribution. Continual peeling skin syndrome is familial and is characterized by large sheets of skin that can be removed intact without causing trauma. Desquamation is generalized but spares the palms and soles. The disorder persists for life.

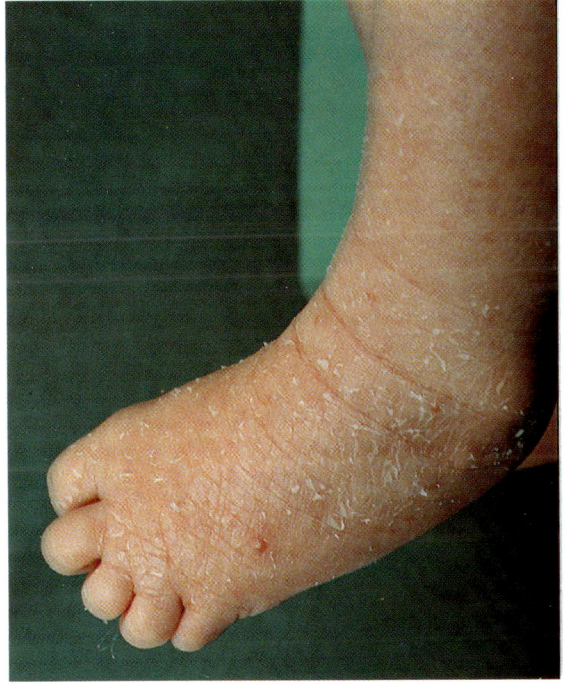

Figure 5.1

Physiological scaling of the newborn. This desquamation is frequently localized to the ankles and feet, and is characterized by noninflammatory, thin scales. It is usually more evident in postmature infants.

DIGITAL ABNORMALITIES

Polydactyly consists of a rudimentary supernumerary digit present at birth. The most common site is near the base of the fifth toe.

Syndactyly is the partial or complete fusion of two digits, usually the second and the third toes. It may be observed in hamartomatous disorders, such as Proteus syndrome, or genetically determined diseases, such as oral-facial-digital syndrome or ectodermal dysplasias.

Megalodactyly is the massive enlargement of the digits. Broad toes, usually the first toe, may be seen in Proteus syndrome or Rubinstein–Taybi syndrome (mental retardation, characteristic facial features, a tendency to form keloids and megalodactyly).

Brachydactyly means shortness of the fingers and toes. It may be seen in ectodermal dysplasias, such as oral-facial-digital syndrome and oculodentodigital dysplasias.

Clinodactyly is the congenital inward bending of a digit, most commonly the fifth toe.

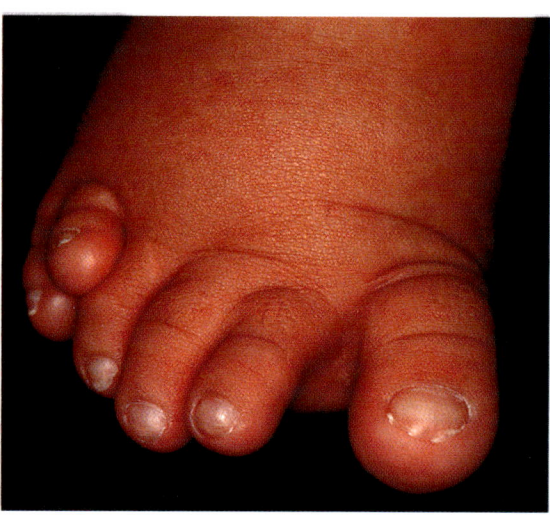
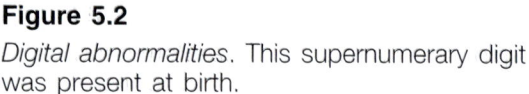

Figure 5.2
Digital abnormalities. This supernumerary digit was present at birth.

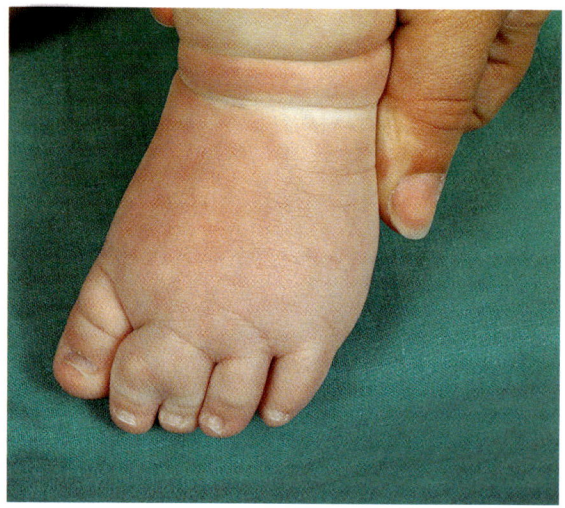

Figure 5.3
Digital abnormalities: syndactyly. Partial fusion of the second and third toe in a patient with Proteus syndrome.

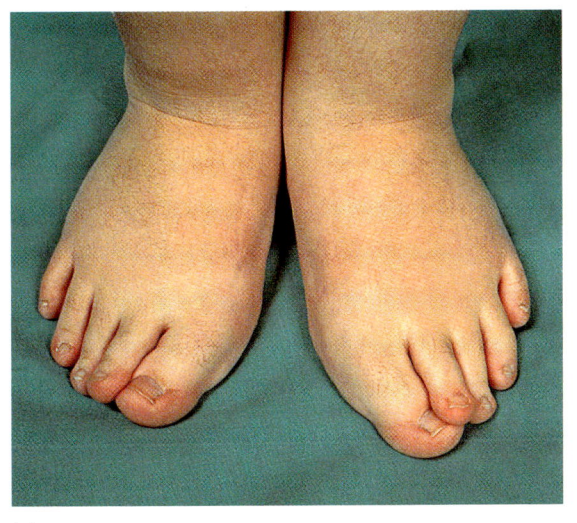
(a)

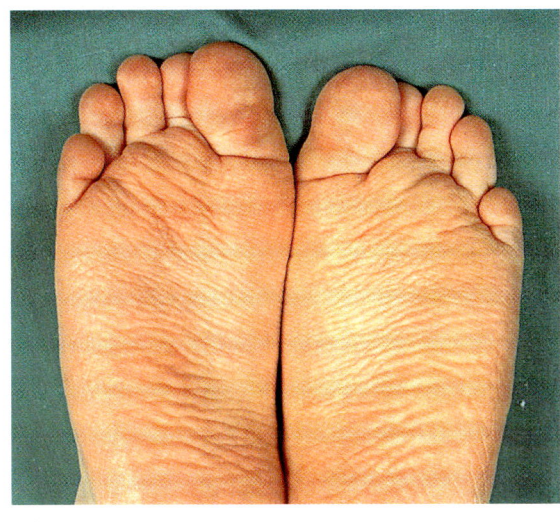
(b)

Figure 5.4
Digital abnormalities: megalodactyly. This first toe may be broad in dysplasia syndromes.

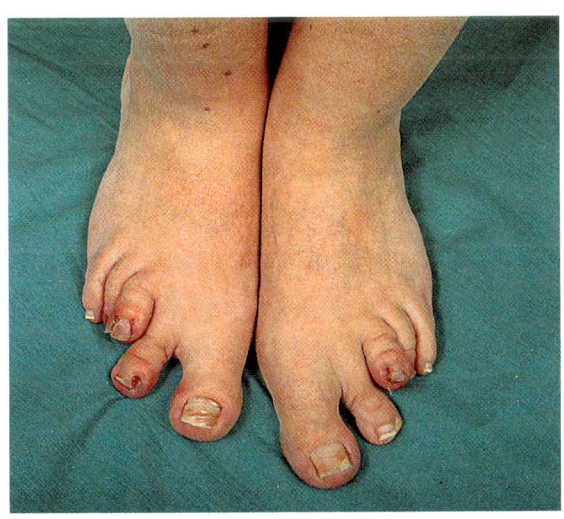

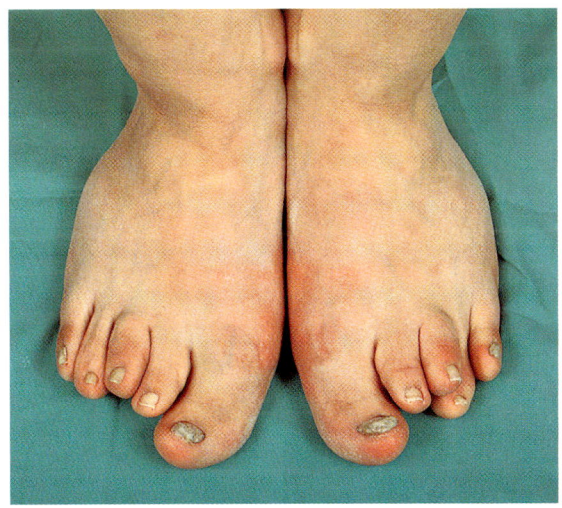

Figure 5.5
Digital abnormalities: brachydactyly. The third, fourth and fifth toes of this patient with orofacial-digital syndrome are short.

Figure 5.6
Digital abnormalities: clinodactyly. Clinodactyly indicates the congenital inward-bending of a toe.

PRIMARY CUTANEOUS LOCALIZED AMYLOIDOSIS

Two forms of primary cutaneous amyloidosis have been described on feet: the papular form (lichen amyloidosus) and the nodular form.

In lichen amyloidosus the lesions consist of persistent, pruritic, firm, nonelastic, nontender, hyperkeratotic, closely set, pea-sized, skin-coloured or brownish dome-shaped or hemispheric papules. In this form the pretibial area is the site most commonly affected. The ankles and the dorsal aspect of the feet are sometimes severely affected.

The nodular form is extremely rare and involves bilaterally the sole. This assumes a waxy, bosselated appearance.

Histologically, the lesions of both forms consist of a deposition of amyloid in the papillary and mid-dermis.

Differential diagnosis

Lichen planus hypertrophicus tends to be verrucous and violaceous in outline; mucous membrane lesions may be present.

Lichen myxoedematosus and lichen simplex chronicus need histological examination.

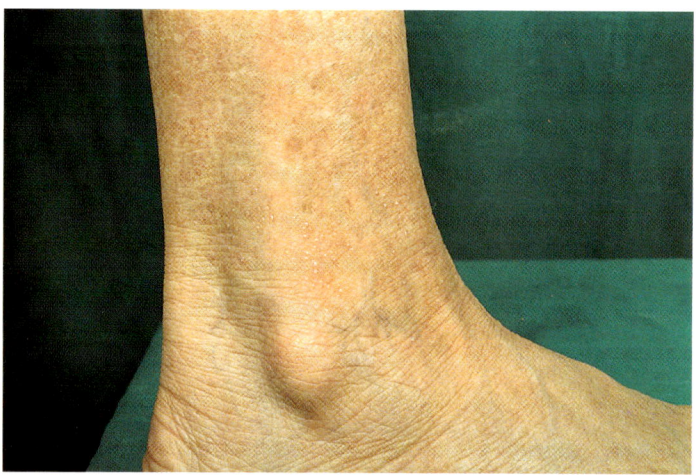

Figure 5.7

Primary cutaneous localized amyloidosis: lichen amyloidosus. Hyperkeratotic, skin-coloured, closely set, firm papules are evident on the ankle and the back of the foot. These lesions are extremely pruritic.

GOUT

Gout is a metabolic disorder characterized by recurrent attacks of acute arthritis that involves preferentially the joints of the lower extremities; hyperuricaemia; and the deposition of needle-shaped crystals of monosodium urates in the articular cartilage and in the skin (tophi). Histologically, tophi consist of an inflammatory reaction around deposits of needle-shaped crystals of monosodium urate, which are readily detected under polarized light.

Clinical features

Acute gouty arthritis usually involves the joints of the lower extremities. It most frequently affects the great toe, which appears warm, red and tender, mimicking acute cellulitis. When the acute attack subsides, the skin becomes violaceous in colour and desquamation appears. In chronic forms, subcutaneous tophi, mainly located on the toes, have a characteristic mottled, salmon-pink colour. Large tophi may spontaneously drain an amber fluid containing crystals of monosodium urate.

Differential diagnosis

Bacterial cellulitis is ruled out by the absence of hyperuricaemia, the presence of fever and lymphangitis, and the prompt response to antibiotics.

Chondrocalcinosis (pseudogout) may be easily diagnosed by X-ray.

Xanthomatous lesions and papules of multicentric reticulohistiocytosis may be differentiated from tophi histologically.

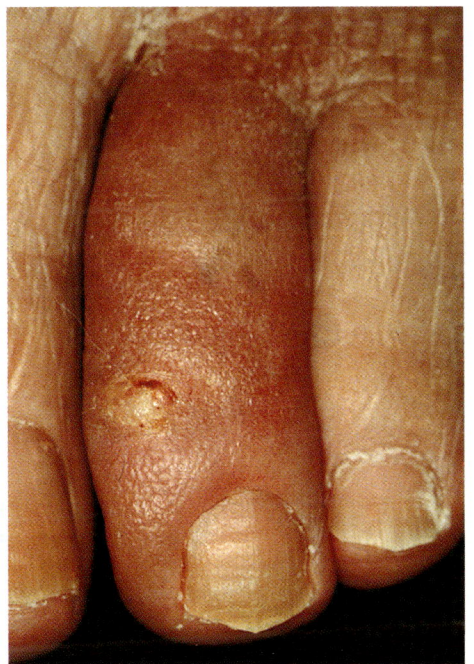

Figure 5.8
Gout. This toe is warm and violaceous presenting with spontaneous damage.

LIPOATROPHY

Lipoatrophy is characterized by the absence of subcutaneous tissue. Two forms of lipoatrophy may involve the feet: lipoatrophy of the ankles and lipoatrophy of Köbberling–Dunnegan.

Lipoatrophy of the ankles is a localized lipoatrophy that manifests as a symmetrical, asymptomatic, depressed band, about 10 cm wide, preceded by noninflammatory swelling of subcutaneous fat.

Lipoatrophy of Köbberling–Dunnegan is a very rare, partial lipoatrophy, usually symmetrical and slowly progressive. It is restricted to the extremities.

Differential diagnosis

Lipoatrophy may be misdiagnosed as scleroderma but, in this disease, the skin is indurated and pearly white.

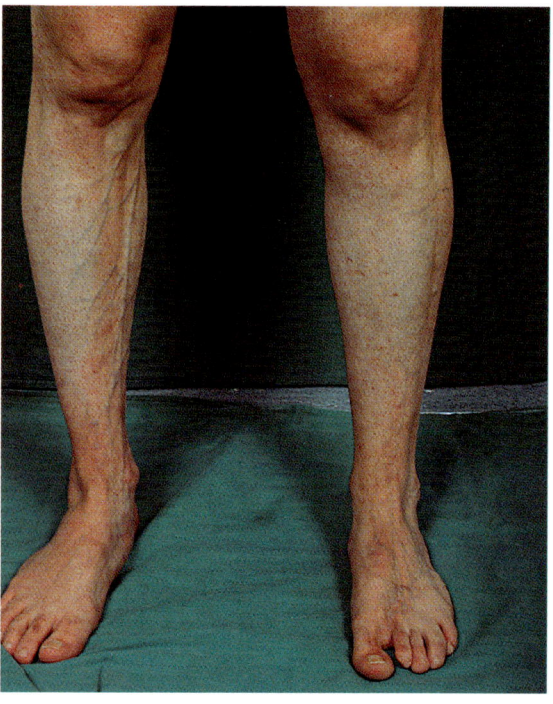

Figure 5.9
Lipoatrophy. A band of lipoatrophy on the dorsum of the foot (Köbberling–Dunnegan type).

PIEZOGENIC PEDAL PAPULES

Piezogenic pedal papules are multiple, soft, skin-coloured protuberances that appear on the posterior part of the medial side of the foot about the heel when weight is placed on the foot. The lesions are usually asymptomatic but may be painful. They most commonly occur in athletes who submit their feet to great stress.

Piezogenic pedal papules are more frequent in the age range 20–30 years. The term 'piezogenic' itself means the induction of papules by pressure (piezo = to press; genic = giving rise to).

The painless papules consist of normal fat tissue. Pain seems to be caused by the herniation of fat into the dermis. The lesions are so characteristic that differential diagnosis is not necessary.

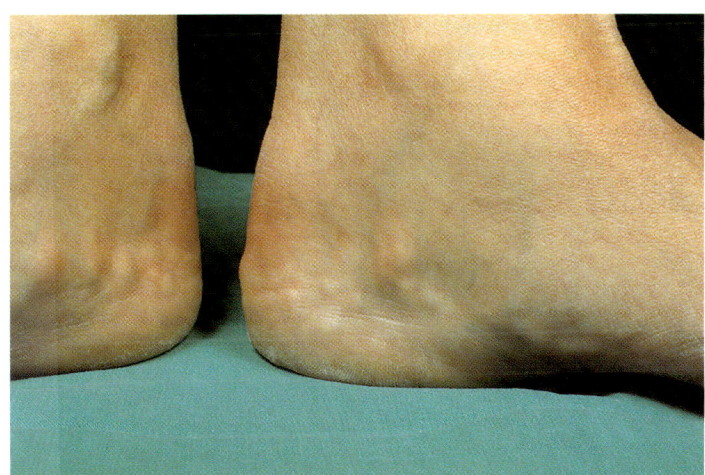

Figure 5.10

Piezogenic pedal papules. This disorder consists of multiple, soft, skin-coloured, asymptomatic protuberances that appear at the posterior aspect of the medial side of the feet above the heel when weight is placed on the feet.

PARANEOPLASTIC ACROKERATOSIS

Paraneoplastic acrokeratosis (or Bazex's syndrome) is characterized by acral and symmetrical cutaneous lesions. It is associated with an underlying internal malignancy.

The cutaneous findings consist of papulo-squamous lesions, hyperpigmentation, parony-chia, nail dystrophy and keratoderma.

The most common associated malignancy is squamous cell carcinoma of the upper digestive tract.

Clinical features

The cutaneous manifestations develop gradually, initially with a characteristic blue to violaceous erythema with peripheral scaling on the soles. Subsequently, the lesions become hyperkeratotic and assume the appearance of a psoriatic kerato-derma. Nail dystrophy is often associated with the disorder. The appearance of the cutaneous lesions precedes the diagnosis of the associated malignancy in about 70% of cases. Resolution may occur with successful resection of the tumour.

Differential diagnosis

The associated nail dystrophy means that the disorder must be differentiated from psoriasis and tinea pedis.

Psoriasis of often familial, involves the scalp and lacks the characteristic violaceous erythema present in Bazex's syndrome.

Tinea pedis may be readily ruled out by micro-scopic examination and culture.

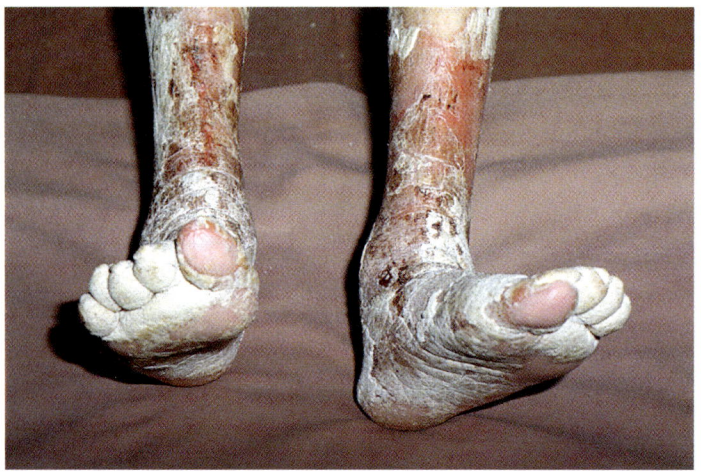

Figure 5.11

Paraneoplastic acrokeratosis: Bazex's syndrome. This symmetrical, psoriatic keratoderma was associated with a carcinoma of the oesophagus.

LIVEDO RETICULARIS

Livedo reticularis is an asymptomatic, cyanotic discolouration of the skin that has a characteristic network-like pattern. The colour of the cyanotic areas is a consequence of the dilatation of the capillaries and small venules. The livedo reticularis pattern is frequently found on the legs, but rarely on the dorsal aspect of the feet. In addition to the physiological form that is linked to exposure to the cold (cutis marmorata), there are two other primary forms: cutis marmorata telangiectatica congenita and idiopathic livedo reticularis with systemic involvement (Sneddon's syndrome).

Cutis marmorata telangiectatica congenita is a congenital, usually asymmetrical, reticulated vascular network, bluish-violet in colour, of unknown aetiology. The areas of skin enclosed by the reticulated pattern may be normal or erythematous. Atrophy of the skin enclosed by the reticulated pattern may be normal or erythematous. Atrophy of the skin and subcutis, and ulcerations of the reticulated bands, are characteristic features. This uncommon vascular anomaly frequently fades with time but may be associated with other congenital malformations.

Idiopathic livedo reticularis with systemic involvement (Sneddon's syndrome) occurs during the third or fourth decade of life, particularly on the limbs. It is associated with coronary, renal and cerebral arterial disease. Prognosis is poor. Laboratory tests do not reveal antinuclear or anticardiolipin antibodies.

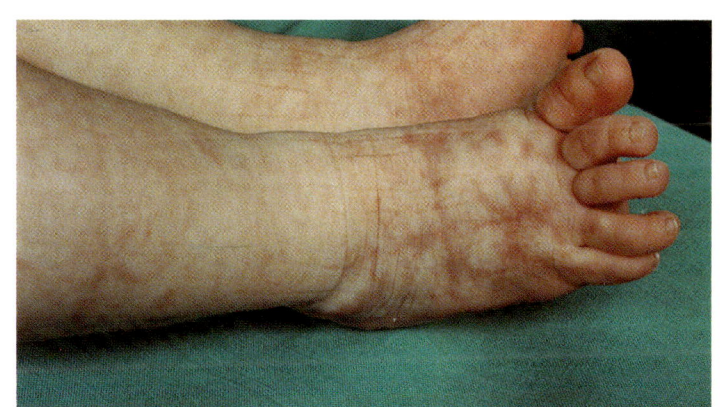

Figure 5.12

Livedo reticularis: cutis marmorata telangiectatica congenita. This congenital, reticular, vascular network, bluish violet in colour, involves the back of a foot. It is associated with atrophy of the subcutis.

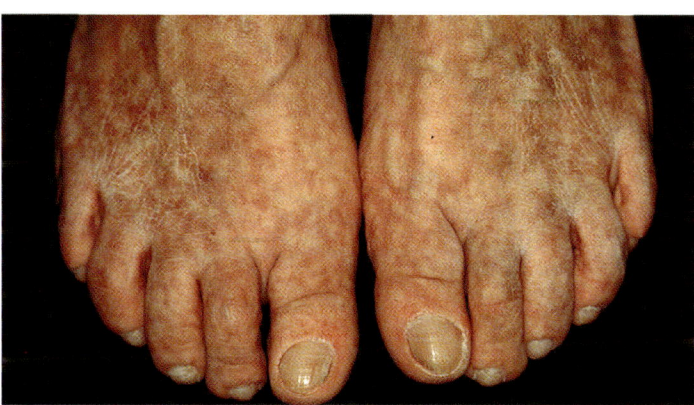

Figure 5.13

Livedo reticularis with systemic involvement: Sneddon's syndrome. This unusual pattern on the dorsal aspect of the feet occurred in the fourth decade of life in a patient with coronary and renal disease. (Photograph courtesy of Professor Antonella Tosti.)

VENOUS ULCERS

Venous ulcers are very frequent trophic lesions with a chronic course of progression. They are usually located on the distal third of the leg, on the internal face or sub-malleolar region.

They are caused by an orthostatic venous hypertension secondary to valvular incompetence of the superficial veins (great and/or small saphenous vein), perforating veins or deep iliac-femoral-popliteal veins. In this last instance the insufficiency is a consequence of deep venous thrombosis; in the others it is a consequence of varicose veins.

There is no pain if there is no bacterial infection. The disease progresses in a typical fashion. In all varicosities (although in different ways) the first sign of venous stasis appears as haemosiderin pigmentation, which then progresses to Milian's white atrophy. Inside this involved area the ulcer opens, often following hidden trauma. Prognosis is dependent upon the appropriate treatment, which is based on three principles: sterilization (if clinical signs of infection are present), surgical, pharmacological or hydrocolloid-based detersion and, lastly, compression with an elastic compressive bandage. Steady resolution of the ulcer will be achieved, if possible, with surgical suppression of the reflux in the saphenous and/or perforating veins. If resolution is not possible or in cases of post-thrombotic syndrome, treatment is based upon a therapeutic elastic stocking.

Clinical features

The essential clinical findings are oedema, cyanosis, varicose veins or previous deep venous thrombosis, pigmentation and white atrophy. On the foot the signs of an orthostatic venous stasis are small, branching veins, isolated or diffuse, in the form of Van der Molen's corona phlebectatica. Leg ulcers are usually sited at the internal malleolar aspect. They are rarely sited at the external retromalleolar aspect if the small saphenous vein is strongly dilated.

If the ulcer is accompanied by mild varicosities, an insufficient perforating vein at the malleolar site (Cockett's communication perforating veins) should be suspected.

Instrumental vascular diagnosis is very useful. Echo-Doppler examination will reveal evidence that is useful for prognosis and treatment: continence or incontinence or deep veins, saphenous veins and perforating veins. Such a procedure has completely replaced plethysmographies and invasive phlebography.

Ischaemic lesions secondary to atherosclerosis or thromboangitis obliterans initially appear at the most distal sites: the digits. As a result of decubitus they also frequently appear in the calcaneus. As association with venous hypertension is possible, but rare. In such cases previous intermittent claudication must be established by investigation in the patient's history. Arterial pulses must be examined and, lastly, an echo-Doppler exam will confirm the diagnosis. Clinically the signs of both pathologies are present.

Hypertensive ischaemic ulcers have different clinical characteristics. These are located at the external malleolar aspect instead of the internal malleolar aspect. These ulcers are typically painful and often surrounded by a cyanotic, reddish zone. Varices are absent.

Arteriovenous fistula: in the congenital forms of this disorder, there is an increase in the length and circumference of the limb, haemangiomas, cyanosis and atypical diffused varicosities.

In cases of localized post-traumatic arteriovenous fistula, the patient will be able to recall a penetrating injury. The trophic lesion is distal and is usually located on the foot. A thrill and a bruit at the tibial artery will be noticed by the patient. The veins are dilated. An echo-Doppler examination will reveal the typical haemodynamic changes: reduction of peripheral resistencies in the artery, arterial pulse in the vein.

Diabetic foot: this trophic lesion is found at different sites distally and at the soles. The possibility of necrobiosis lipoidica must be considered. An association between a venous ulcer and diabetes mellitus is not uncommon, which results in a worsening of the prognosis and the necessity to treat both pathologies.

Ulcers of erythema induratum are usually found in the lateral or posterior side of the lower leg. These are often bilateral and symmetrical. Varicosities, oedema and signs of venous stasis are absent.

Trophic lesions secondary to vasculitis, scleroderma or cryoglobulinaemia often have a morphology similar to a venous ulcer. Frequently located at malleolar sites, these are often bilateral and numerous.

Carcinomatous ulcers: a frequently encountered tumour is squamous cell carcinoma that may grow on a pre-existing venous ulcer (called, in this case, Marjolin's ulcer). Such tumours must be suspected if the ulcer has hard, elevated margins.

Basal-cell carcinoma is also encountered. This, too, may be observed at the internal malleolar aspect but is not as similar in appearance to a venous ulcer as is a squamous cell carcinoma.

In both cases definitive diagnosis will be established by histology.

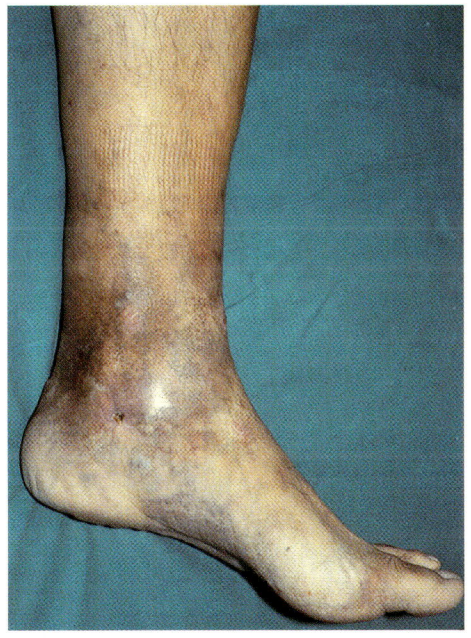

Figure 5.14

Early venous ulcer. An early venous ulcer located typically at the internal malleolar aspect. Clinical signs of chronic venous stasis are evident at the distal third of the leg and on the foot. There is no evidence of veins on the leg. This is more commonly secondary to deep venous thrombosis than to varicose veins. Patient history and a venous echo-Doppler will help to establish the aetiology.

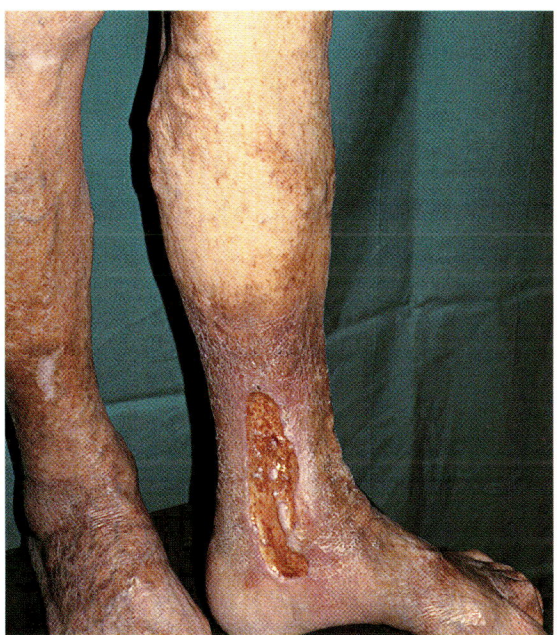

Figure 5.15

Advanced venous ulcer at a typical site. Clinical examination demonstrates evident truncal varices along the aspect of the great saphenous vein, which explains the ulcer's aetiology. The diffuse haemosiderin pigmentation is secondary to chronic venous hypertension.

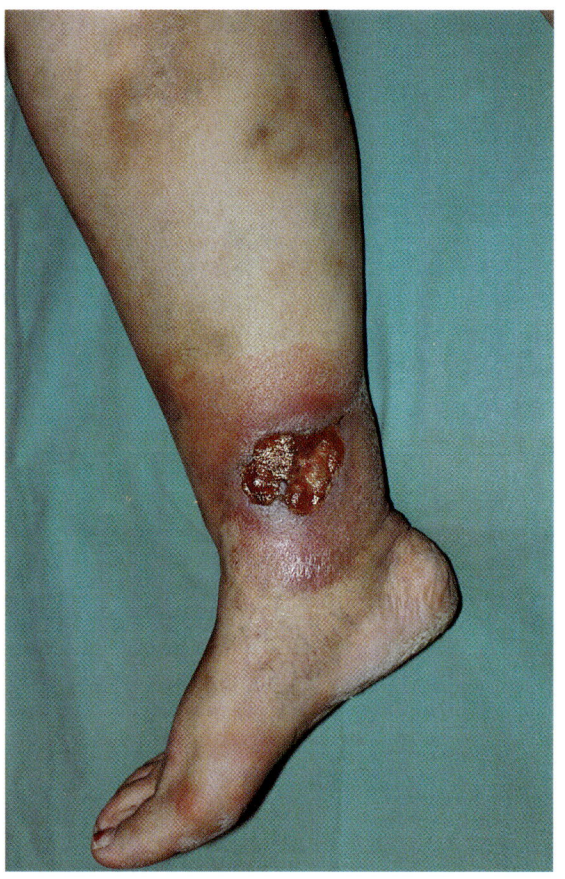

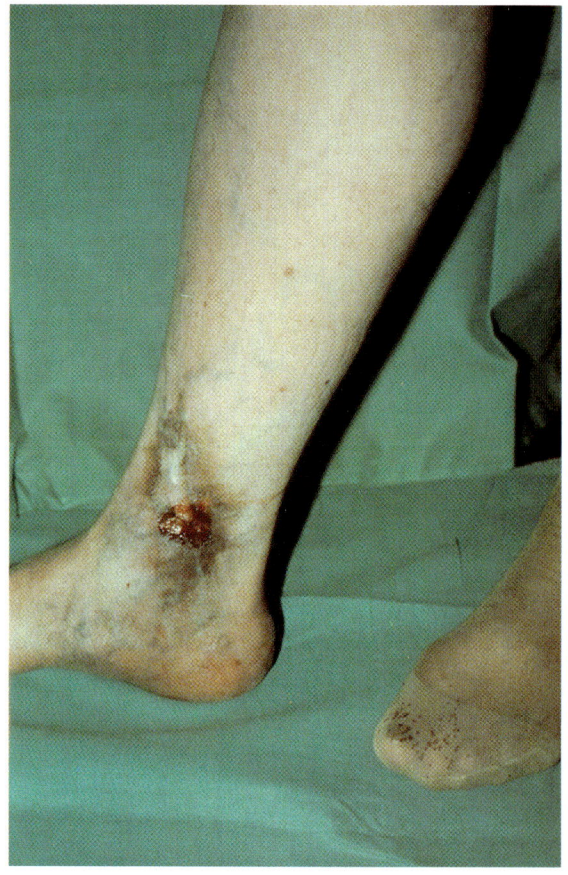

Figure 5.16

Venous ulcer surrounded by reddish oedematous skin. Local pain is present. These features are secondary to significant bacterial infection (in this case *Escherichia coli*).

Figure 5.17

Bleeding venous ulcer with white atrophy and pigmentation. Venous ulcer surrounded by white atrophy and, externally, by pigmentation. No varices are present. Two years previously, the patient suffered a post-partum deep venous thrombosis. The ulcer was induced by a very dilated Cockett's perforator. For this reason the absence of varices does not correlate with the severity of the venous hypertension. The patient presented at the emergency unit of the author's hospital with sudden haemorrhage. This is a common complication of venous ulcers, which can be secondary to minimal trauma or even spontaneous.

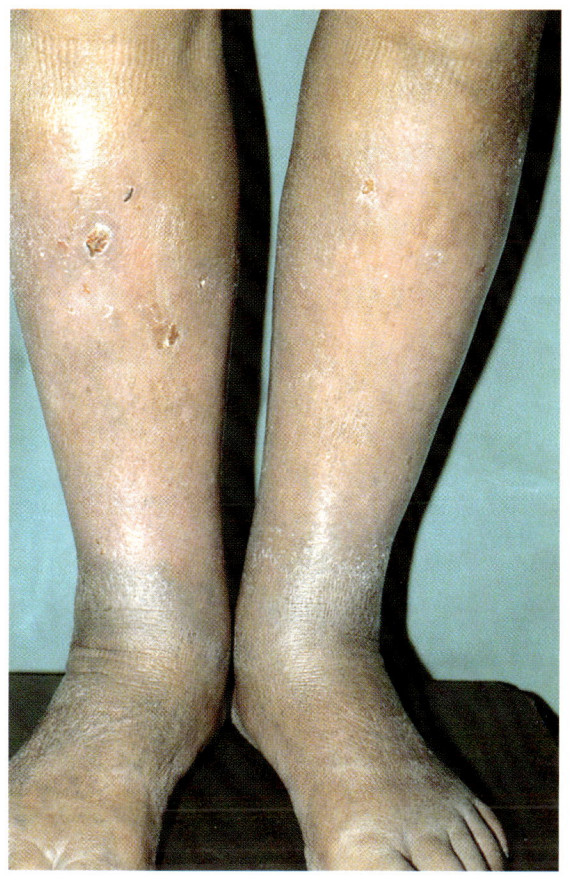

Figure 5.18

Venous hypertension. The presence of varicose veins is not a precondition of venous hypertension. This 48-year old female has oedema and cyanosis secondary to severe venous stasis without varices. She also had a congenital, familial incontinence with reflux in the deep venous system.

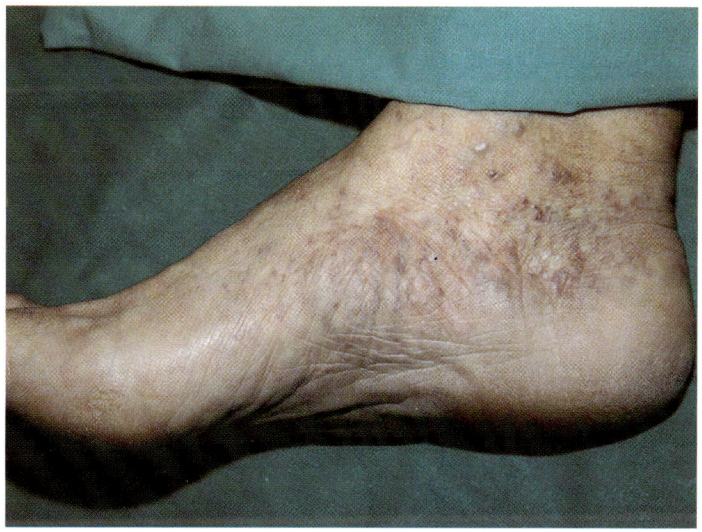

Figure 5.19

Venous ulcer. Diffuse branches of small veins are distributed typically on the foot, with a clinical picture of Van der Molen's corona phlebectatica.

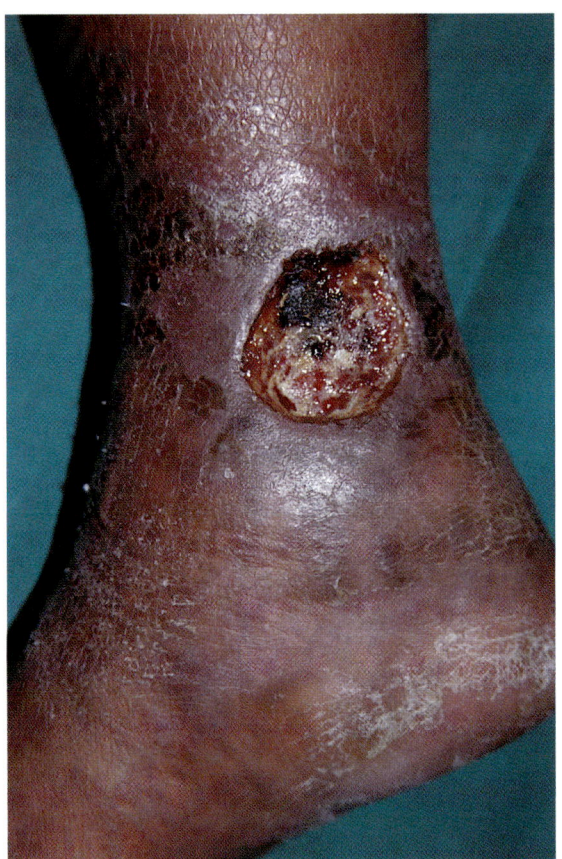

Figure 5.20

Venous ulcer and chronic diabetes mellitis. The foot and the ulcer have the clinical appearance of both pathologies.

ATHEROSCLEROTIC ISCHAEMIC LESIONS

Atherosclerotic arteriopathy is a chronic progressive disease often located in the lower limbs. It is the primary cause of death through myocardial ischaemia. Over 90% of arterial ischaemic lesions in the foot are secondary to atherosclerosis. Trophic lesions are the consequence of a chronic reduction in blood flow and are generally located, in the early stage of the disease, at the ends of the digits, around the nails or in the interdigital spaces. They are also common over bony metatarsal prominences due to compression of the shoes, and on the heel as a result of the pressure caused by feet resting on the bed. Clinical characteristics include the tendency to spread to the proximal aspect of the foot. The base of the initial lesion is grey, yellowish or black as a consequence of necrosis.

The surrounding skin is cyanotic or reddish and never normal. The foot's skin is cold. Granulation is absent. The prognosis in treated patients is connected with a low tendency to epithelization. Osteomyelitis may necessitate amputation. Tendon exposure is frequent and rapid.

Clinical features

Atherosclerotic necrosis is the last stage in the evolution of a chronic disease. It is typically preceded by intermittent claudication and then by pain when at rest.

Arterial tibial pulses are absent while these may be present in embolic and diabetic ischaemia. Leg muscles are atrophic. Hair does not grow on the dorsal aspect of the toes and foot.

The diagnosis is clinical. An echo-Doppler is useful in obtaining morphological and haemodynamic information – the first to show the site and extent of the main stenosis and occlusions; the second to show the severity and possible prognosis of the disease, and to chart the disease's evolution and the efficacy of treatment.

Differential diagnosis

Diabetes can induce trophic lesions on the digits, but other typical sites are on the soles, the heels and the distal aspect of the leg. Gangrene is wet, often with bacterial contamination. Local pain is often absent. Previous intermittent claudication is often absent and rest pain in the leg is weaker, if present at all.

Acute embolism on a smaller scale causes limited severe necrosis in the foot. If the thrombus is larger, the occlusion is proximal and the ischaemia extends to the leg.

The onset of pain and clinical evolution are, moreover, very rapid.

Thromboangitis obliterans involves only medium and small-sized arteries, with distal claudication and the rapid onset of trophic lesions. Patients tend to be young males and heavy smokers. Proximal pulses are present. Definitive diagnosis is confirmed by histology.

Venous ulcers are usually located at the internal malleolar aspect and are accompanied by evidence of venous disease. It is possible to observe a mixed ulcer in a patient who has also become atherosclerotic. The symptoms and clinical features arise as a result of the two concomitant pathologies.

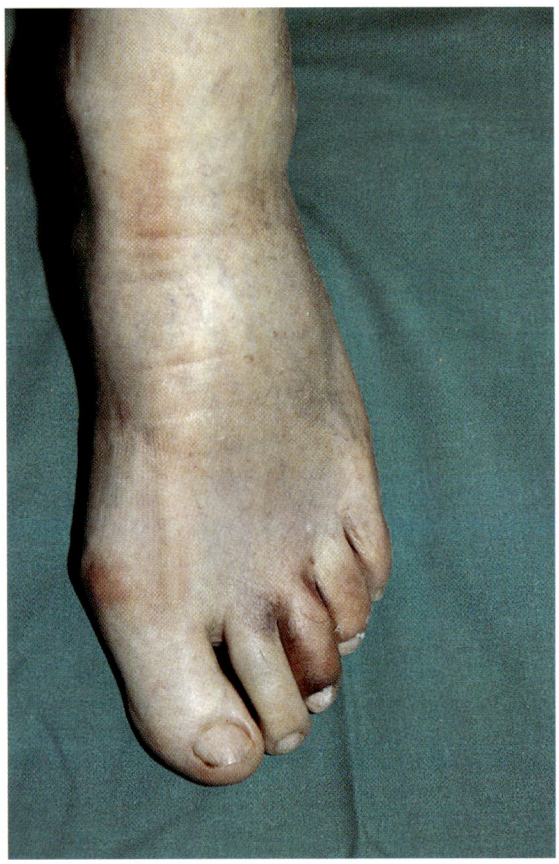

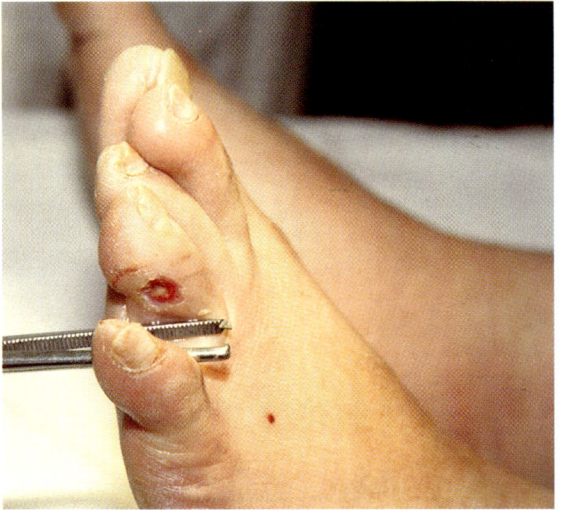

Figure 5.22

Atherosclerotic ischaemia lesions. Early ischaemic trophic lesions located on the surfaces of two contiguous toes. These pressure lesions are called 'kissing ulcers'.

Figure 5.21

Atherosclerotic ischaemic lesions. Initial ischaemic lesions on the foot in a patient affected by long-lasting chronic atherosclerosis that is characterized by progressive worsening of the symptoms through intermittent claudication and rest pain.

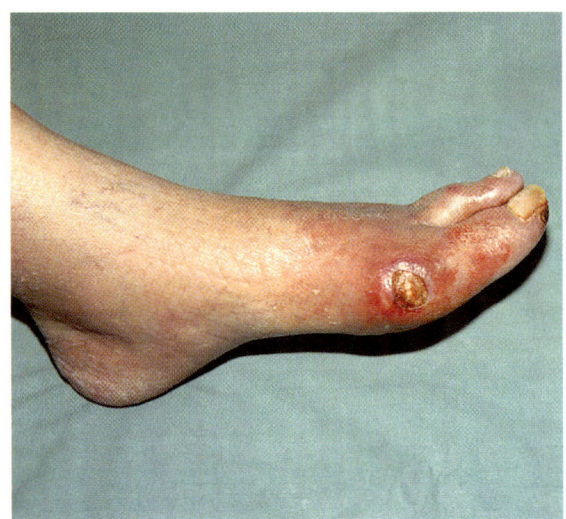

Figure 5.23

Ischaemic lesions secondary to compression by the shoes. The typical site is over the bony metatarsal prominence, which leads to skin compression.

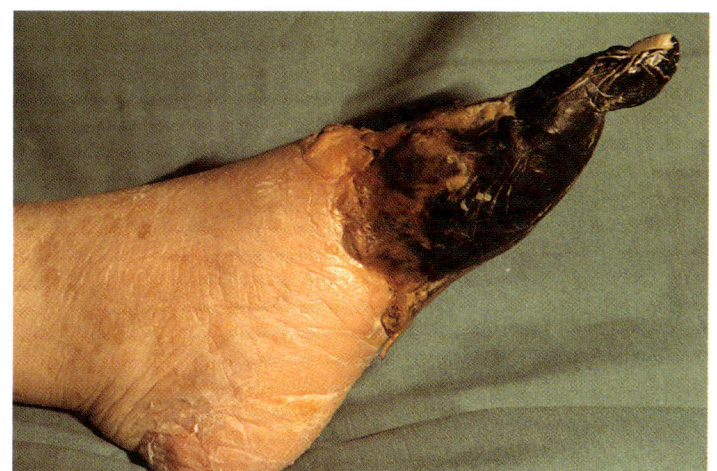

Figure 5.24

Atherosclerotic ischaemic lesions: gangrene of the forefoot. Gangrene secondary to atherosclerosis is, fortunately, often a dry gangrene.

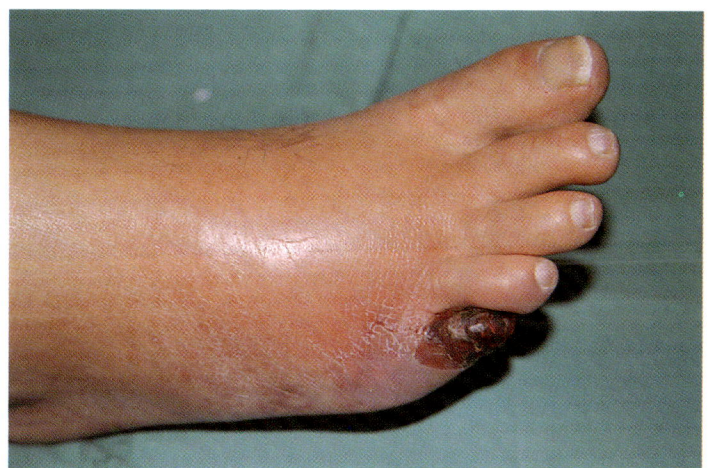

Figure 5.25

Gangrene of a toe secondary to chronic atherosclerotic ischaemia. Chronic, diffuse involvement of the skin is demonstrated by evident changes in the periulcerative tissues, which are reddish, cyanotic and cold. Pain is severe. The gangrene usually spreads spontaneously.

DIABETIC FOOT

Dermal changes secondary to diabetes mellitus are frequent. These are connected with macro- and microangiopathy and with neuropathy. They are always complications of long-standing diabetes. In the relationship between diabetes and trophic lesions, two different scenarios arise. First, the patient may have a macroangiopathy in the form of an atherosclerotic disease, where diabetes is one of the risk factors relevant for therapy and prognosis. Second, there is the case of patient where diabetes has induced diffuse severe microangiopathy with or without macroangiopathy. This situation can, in itself, cause severe necrotic lesions, possibly concomitant with troubles secondary to the macroangiopathy.

When compared to the purely atherosclerotic patient, the diabetic patient is younger. Female prevalence is higher by a ratio of 1:2.

Correct management of hyperglycaemia is necessary but not particularly useful in aiding the resolution of the trophic lesions. The prognosis of diabetic trophic lesions is very variable, and spontaneous healing is possible. Unlike atherosclerotic lesions or any lesions secondary to macroangiopathy, microvascular gangrene of the digits can be treated fairly successfully by amputation. In other cases the gangrene spreads towards the leg. In this instance, the course of the disease is different from atherosclerosis. In diabetes, the distal gangrene is often not complete, sparing one or more digits and extending only partially to the foot and leg. The gangrene's distribution sometimes corresponds to the distribution of the nerves, which confirms the correlation between nervous impairment and tissue necrosis. The gangrene is often wet, which influences its development. Sometimes, therefore, it can develop rapidly and facilitates the growth of bacterial infection that can extend to the tendons and bone.

Necrobiosis lipoidica diabeticorum (NLD) is a rare condition suggesting occult diabetes. The clinical lesions are generally not on the foot but rather on the leg, usually on the anterior aspect.

Clinical features

It is possible to distinguish macro- and microvascular trophic lesions by their clinical appearance. Macrovascular ulcers have the characteristics of atherosclerotic ulcers (distal, painful, with previous intermitted claudication). The onset of microvascular trophic lesions is preceded by neurological changes: hypoaesthesia and deep hyporeflectivity. For this reason, the ulcers are often not painful. The involvement of the vasa nervorum, concomitant to that of the vasa vasorum, is also connected with the localization of the early lesions which are secondary to inapparent microtrauma mainly due to the shoes. Typical sites are the sole, the base of the first digit and the heel. A reactive hyperkeratosis may precede the ulcer, which will have a hard, callous edge. Other initial characteristics are the involvement of the nail-bed and bacterial or fungal infection that sometimes leads to the spontaneous loss of the nail. Tibial pulses may be present which proves there is no macrovascular involvement.

Lastly, hyposensitivity of the foot is common but hyperaesthetic with strong pain and thermal and tactile disaesthesia are also possible.

Serum glycaemia is the benchmark in monitoring the patient's metabolic status. The correction of glycaemic values is necessary but usually has no effect on the development of trophic lesions on the foot.

Differential diagnosis

Atherosclerotic chronic ischaemia: pain is present. Arterial tibial pulses are absent. Intermittent claudication always precedes the onset of skin changes. Trophic lesions are at the distal aspect of the digits or secondary to decubitus on the calcaneus.

Acute ischaemia arterial trophic lesions: pain and local symptoms appear suddenly. Pulses are absent at the site of arterial occlusion.

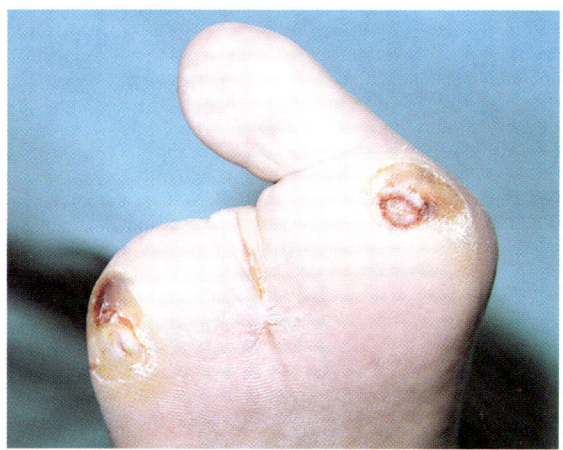

Figure 5.26

A typical diabetic foot. This patient suffered at various times from gangrene of the digits. This was treated with distal amputation, which resulted in complete resolution. Unlike these, trophic lesions localized at the laying points do not heal. Pressure ulcers appear inside hyperkeratotic, callous skin.

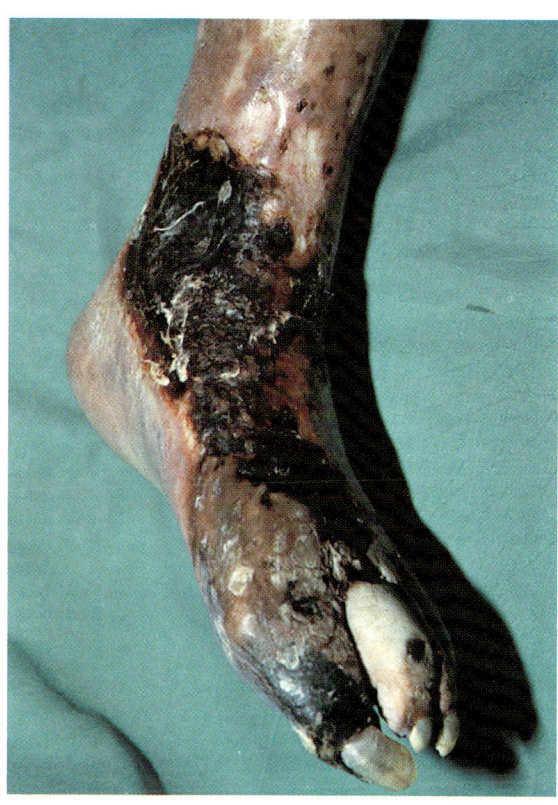

Figure 5.27

Diabetic gangrene of the foot. The gangrene began on the first digit, extended rapidly to the sole of the medial aspect of the foot, and then to the malleolus. It did not involve the other digits and the heel.

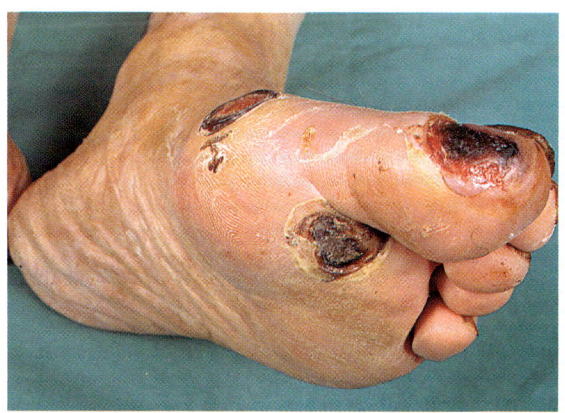

Figure 5.28

Patient with diabetic neuropathy. Decubitus ulcers or pressure sores are frequent in such cases. The lesions result from the prolonged application of pressure from shoes, concentrated in a relatively small area of skin which is microangiopathic. A callus often surrounds and precedes the opening of the lesion.

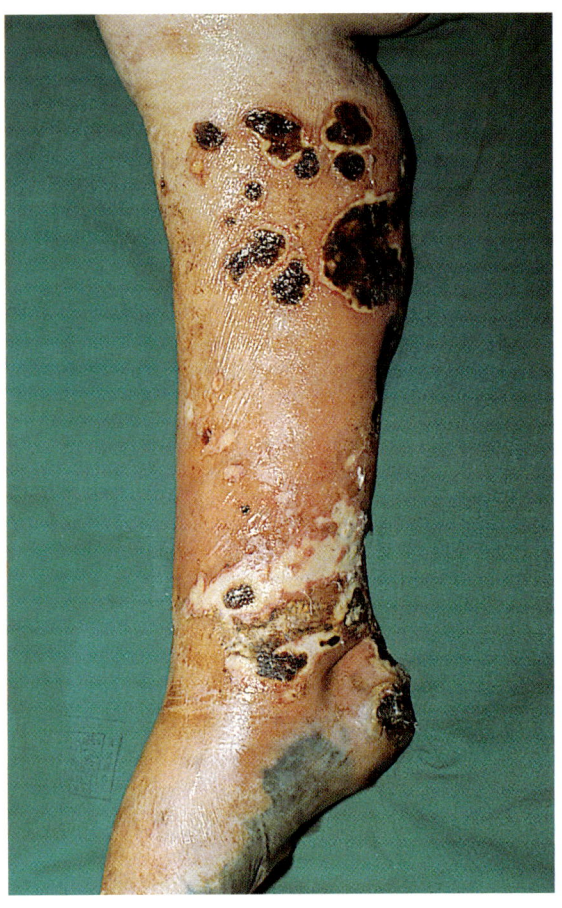

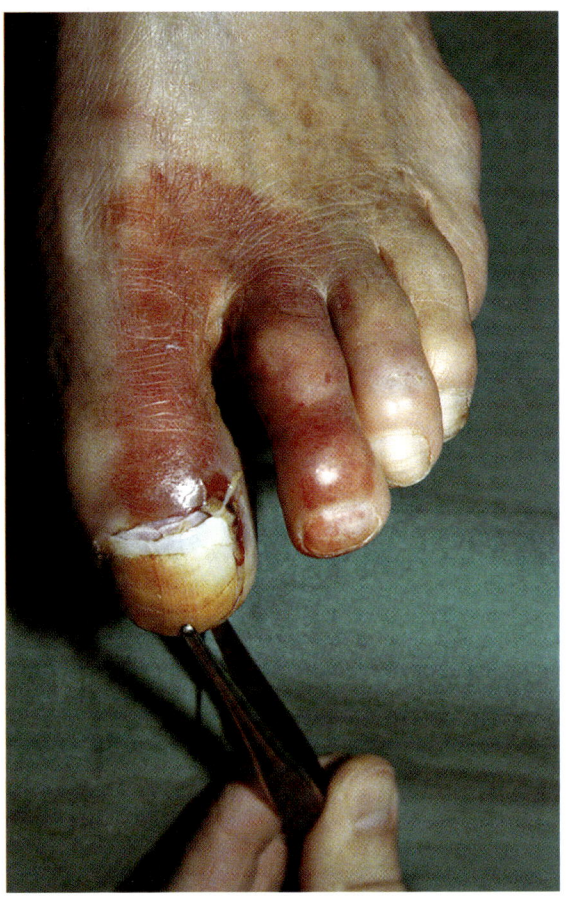

Figure 5.29

Diabetic lesions on the feet and leg. On the sole of the right foot, a recent wide necrosis is accompanied by a previous gangrene located on the heel. Several other necrotic areas can be observed on the leg.

Figure 5.30

Diabetic foot: initial trophic involvement. Initial trophic impairment in a diabetic patient, located at the first and second digits. While the skin is slightly involved, the nail-beds are involved severely, with spontaneous detachment of the nail.

LYMPHOEDEMA

Lymphoedema is swelling of the foot (sometimes extending to the limb and thigh) secondary to the accumulation of lymph. Primary lymphoedema may be congenital and may appear at puberty (praecox) or after the age of 35 (tardum), and is usually bilateral.

Secondary lymphoedema is the result of infection, chronic inflammation, neoplastic involvement of the nodes, radiotherapy and/or (less frequently) the surgical ablation of the lymph nodes.

Lymphatic stasis in the tissue, whatever the cause, leads to protein deposition in the interstitial spaces, fibroblastic proliferation and the formation of connective tissue. Clinically, the soft oedema becomes a hard oedema. Episodes of secondary infections have been reported in about 20% of cases.

Clinical features

The initial symptom is a puffiness at the dorsal aspect of the foot and in the ankle region; this oedema increased at the end of the day.

With the increase of the oedema, a characteristic lump appears on the dorsal aspect of the foot in the form of a 'pin cushion'. This swelling reduces only slightly during a period of prolonged rest in bed. Digital compression does not reduce oedema any more. The foot, and then the limb and thigh, become very large, unsightly and heavy, but without pain. Extensive fibrosis of the subcutaneous tissue appears at the distal aspect of the limb.

Ulceration of the foot or leg is usually secondary to trauma. Lymphorrhoea is frequent. There is no pain if there is no infection. Granulation quickly becomes evident. Healing depends on the possibility of correcting the oedema with compression.

In very advanced cases, the epidermis becomes hyperkeratotic and warty, giving the legs and feet an elephantiasis-like appearance.

The vascular laboratory diagnosis is the only one involved in the instrumental differential diagnosis. An echo-Doppler examination will help in detecting a venous disease that is the consequence of venous reflux or venous thrombosis.

Differential diagnosis

Venous stasis: when secondary to varicose disease, varices are present. If the venous disease is a deep venous thrombosis, oedema develops rapidly with pain and functional impairment. In venous disease, oedema involves the leg and thigh. The foot is only minimally involved, and only in the case of long lasting clinical history. Pain is never present in lymphoedema. Immobility may arise simply as a consequence of the limbs dimensions.

Lipoedema is an augmented thickness of the fatty tissue from the waist down to the ankle. The foot is not involved. This condition is often mistaken for lymphoedema. Lipoedema affects women, is bilateral and symmetrical.

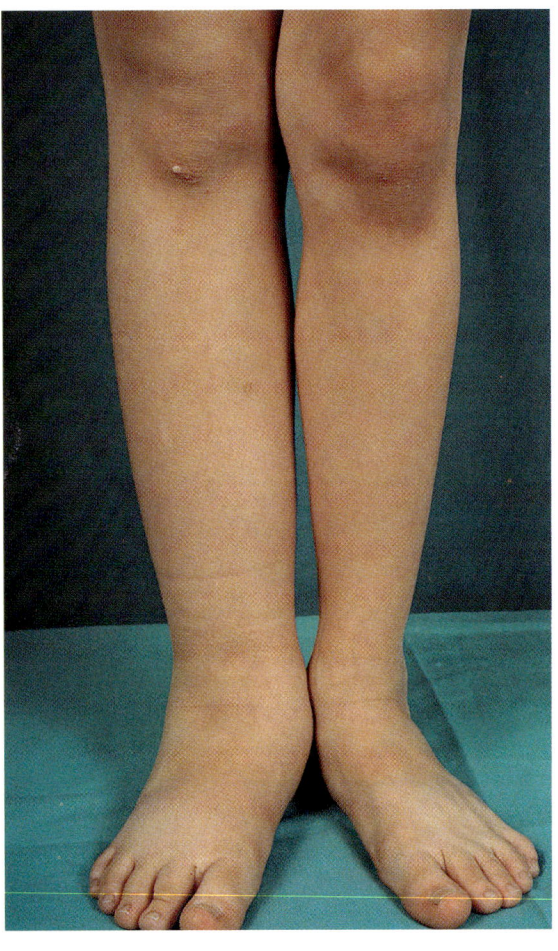

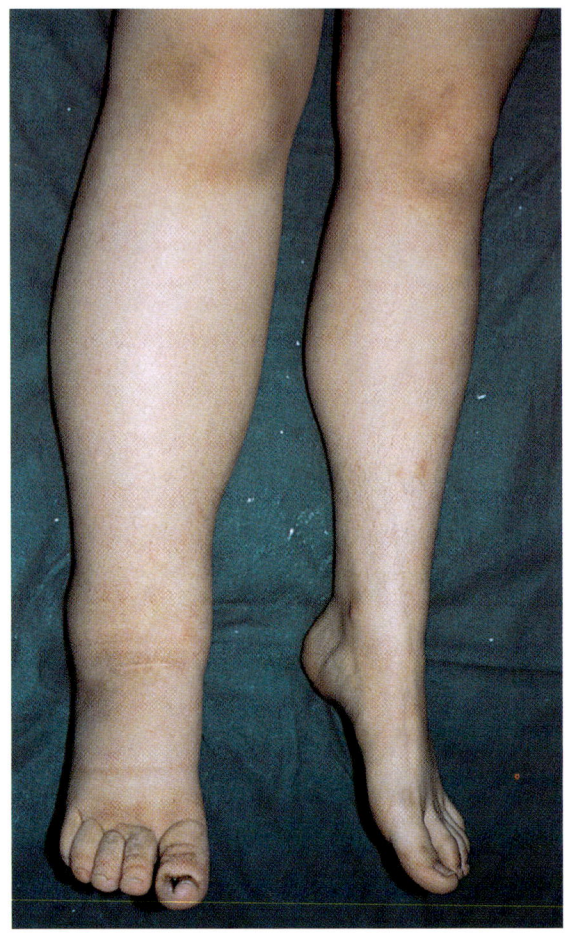

Figure 5.31

Primary lymphoedema. This case of lymphoedema praecox appeared at the age of 3 years.

Figure 5.32

Unilateral lymphoedema. Unilateral lymphoedema with swelling of the foot that has extended to the limb. Infection of the nail-bed of the first digit is common as bacteria grows readily in these protein-rich tissues. Lymphangitis is also frequent. Wounds, abrasions, cuts or nail cuts can be the means of ingress of the bacteria.

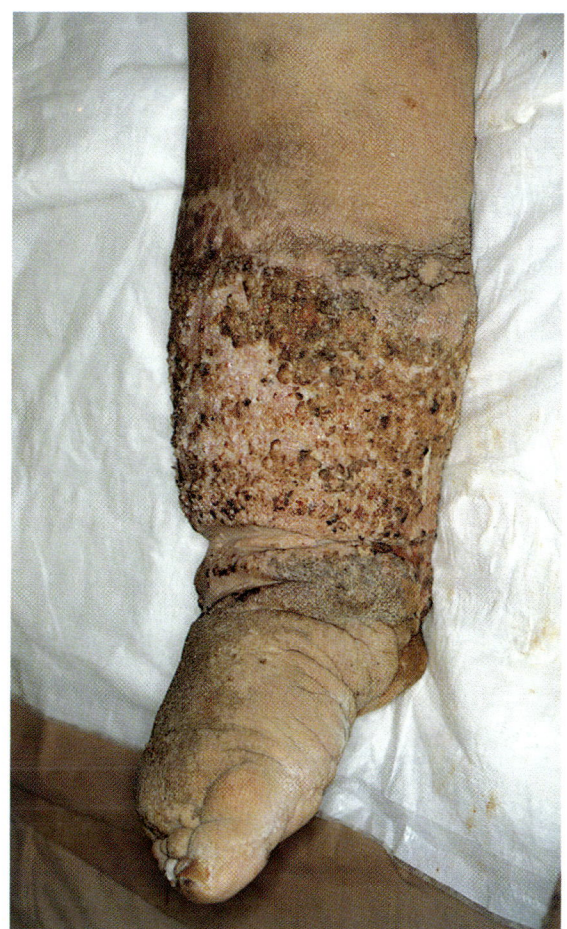

Figure 5.33

Lymphoedema. Lymphoedema is characterized by the presence of keratotic vegetating lesions and papillomatosis.

HYPERTENSIVE ULCERS

Chronic, severe arterial hypertension can develop into an ulcer. Although rare, this condition can be managed with correct antihypertensive therapy. The ulcer appears in an area of bluish skin that is typically located at the distal third of the external aspect of the ankle. The ulcer's base rapidly becomes necrotic and has a very weak tendency to granulation.

In chronic, severe hypertension there is a generalized increase in the thickness of the arterial wall. Myocytes proliferate, the artery becomes rigid and the lumen narrows, leading to microvascular impairment. The reasons for the typical malleolar location of the disorder are not clear.

Patients affected are women in the fifth to seventh decades of life. The disorder extends progressively and both legs are often involved. If appropriate, pharmacological therapy is prescribed (i.e. drug that lowers peripheral vascular resistance), resolution is quite rapid and stable.

Clinical features

The ulcer is typically painful and it is for this reason that medical help is usually sought. Tibial pulses are present or slightly decreased. A painful ulcer in a woman (at the lateral aspect of the ankle) should raise suspicion of a hypertensive ulcer. Arterial blood pressure confirms the clinical hypothesis. An echo-Doppler examination will help in confirming the morphological patency of the arterial bed. From a haemodynamic point of view, the Doppler complex typically shows parietal stiffness.

Differential diagnosis

Venous ulcers are located at the internal aspect of the ankle. An external location is typical of hypertensive ulcer. In venous ulcers varices are usually present, and there is no pain if there is no bacterial infection. Venous ulcers open as white atrophy surrounded by haemosiderin hyperpigmentation. A venous ulcer has usually a bed with active granulation.

Atherosclerotic ischaemic lesions are located distally, at the digits or on the heel, as a consequence of compression. An ulcer at the malleolar aspect is usually the result of trauma. It must be borne in mind, however, that hypertension is one of the main risk factors for atherosclerosis.

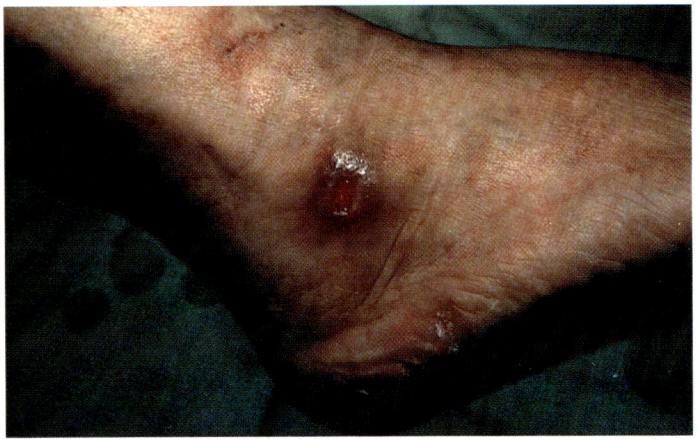

Figure 5.34
Hypertensive ulcer. Hypertensive ulcer typically located at the external aspect of the ankle.

ARTERIOVENOUS FISTULA

The arteriovenous fistula can cause the onset of cutaneous alterations until a real ulcer develops. The blood flows directly from the arterial into the venous bed, resulting in an impairment of peripheral tissue vascularization that causes the trophic lesions.

Congenital arteriovenous fistulas are characterized by an increased length and circumference of the lower limb, and varicose veins on the lateral surface of the thigh in the case of Klippel–Trenaunay–Weber syndrome. In this case, ulcers can appear at various sites but generally at the distal third of the leg.

Arteriovenous traumatic fistulas on the foot are fairly common as a result of injuries by pointed objects at that site. As the fistula evolves, there is often a progressive worsening of the cutaneous microcirculation. In such cases a haemodynamic morphological study of the arteriovenous fistula is necessary (followed by surgical treatment or a venous or arterious embolization).

Clinical features

In congenital arteriovenous fistulas the foot is not frequently involved.

Clinical evaluation must consider the whole limb to demonstrate lengthening of the skeleton and circumference increase, the varicose dilatations and the changing cutaneous trophism in the legs.

The acquired arteriovenous fistulas on the foot are usually the result of injuries by pointed objects. They show signs of trophic cutaneous impairment and of venous hypertension.

Cutaneous pigmentation, hyperkeratosis, papillomatosis of the involved digits and damage to the nail-bed may be observed. The veins on the back of the foot are typically dilated. Arterial pulses are present with hyperpulsatility.

An echo-Doppler examination will help in evaluating vascular haemodynamic changes in a noninvasive manner. The fistula's arterial origin means there will be a reduction in peripherical resistances. The regional veins present a continuous flow with a high velocity and a systolic increase due to the direct blood passage from the arterial bed into the venous bed.

Differential diagnosis

A venous ulcer is typically located at the internal prospect of the malleolus. In this case limbs will be the same length.

In the varicose disorders the varices are mainly in the leg and not in the foot.

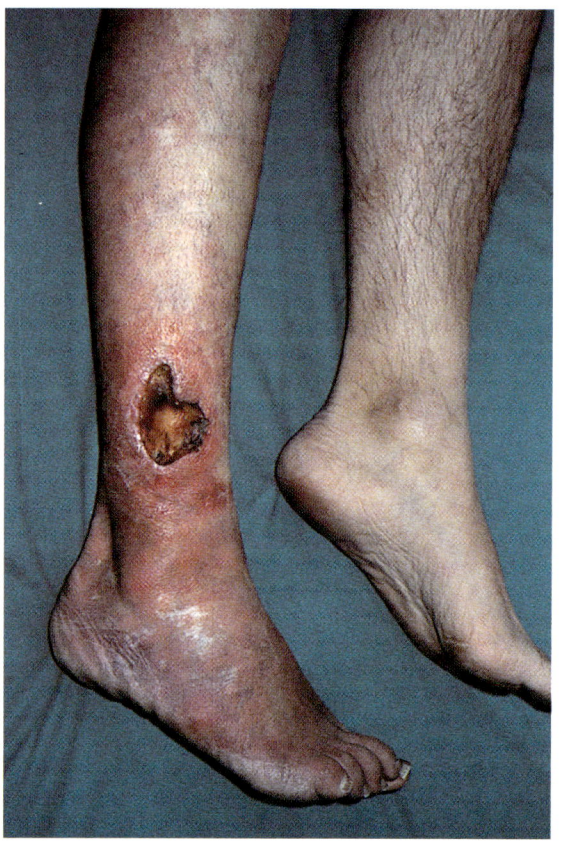 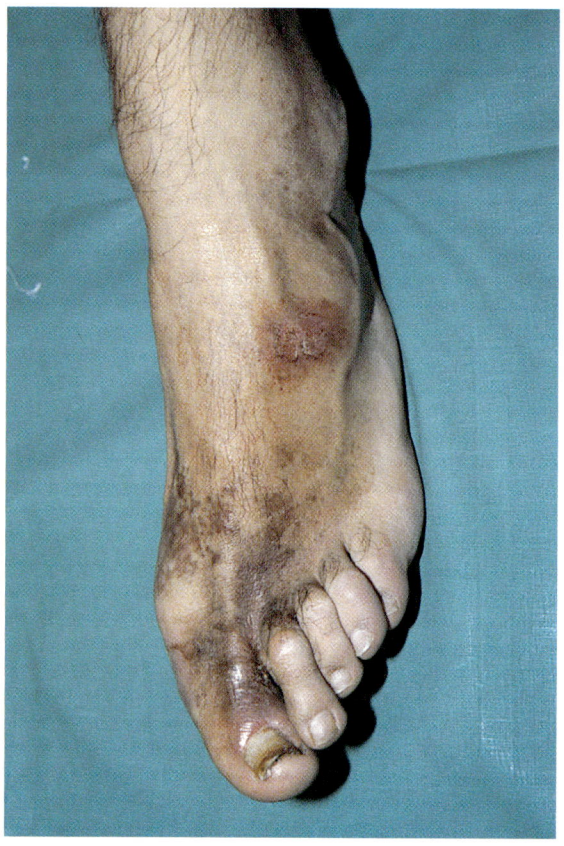

Figure 5.35

Arteriovenous fistula: patient affected by Klippel–Trenaunay syndrome. The affected limb is longer and bigger. Diffuse, telangiectatic areas are present in the leg. A wide ulcer with a fibrous surface and with little tendency to heal is present at the distal external third of the leg.

Figure 5.36

Arteriovenous fistula: in a young male. A recent arteriovenous fistula in a young male, secondary to an accidental knife wound at the base of the fifth metatarsal. Haemosiderin pigmentation, cyanosis and trophic impairment of the first digit, particularly the nail-bed. Regional veins are also evidently dilated in the clinostatic position.

ARTERIAL EMBOLIC ISCHAEMIC LESIONS

A sudden interruption in arterial flow will determine the location of an arterial occlusion. Characteristic symptoms include the acute onset of pain, pallor, a lack of pulses and paraesthesia paralysis as a result of nervous impairment. The embolus can either be of cardiac origin (occluding a normal arterial bed) or of arterial origin (from an atherosclerotic plaque located cranially to the embolized branch).

Clinical features

The skin of the foot is white, cold and painful. Symptoms are always connected with the location of the emboli as well as the presence of the pulses. Arterial echo-Doppler will confirm the diagnosis of arterial occlusion.

Differential diagnosis

Ischaemic chronic atherosclerotic lesions evolve progressively and the onset of trophic lesions always follows the rest pain. Ischaemia, on the other hand, appears suddenly without previous symptoms in cases of emboli of cardiac origin and with acute worsening of previous ischaemic symptoms if the starting point of the emboli is the cranial atherosclerotic arterial tree.

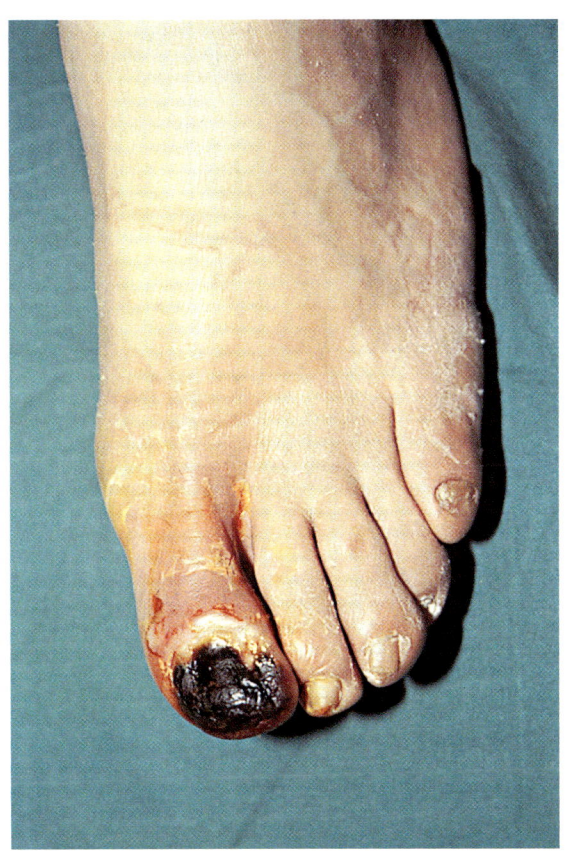

Figure 5.37
Arterial embolic ischaemic lesions. The clinical consequence of a previous arterial embulus in a patient with atrial fibrillation.

CHRONIC PERNIOSIS

Chronic perniosis is, today, a rare cause of trophic lesions in the foot. It appears in the winter and is secondary to arteriospasm. There is complete recovery in periods of warmer weather. The lesions involve the distal aspect of the digits, the dorsal aspect of the feet and the legs. They appear in crops and affect only young women, usually 15–20 years of age.

Differential diagnosis

Atherosclerotic ischaemic chronic lesions are clinically similar. Tibial pulses are absent, while they are present in perniosis. Patients are older. Intermitted claudication and rest pain precede the onset of trophic lesions. In perniosis, lesions appear in winter, with spontaneous recovery in warmer weather.

Clinical features

In the early stage of the disease, multiple, red blisters appear on the toes. The colour then becomes progressively bluish. Finally, the blisters open, leading to painful ulcers.

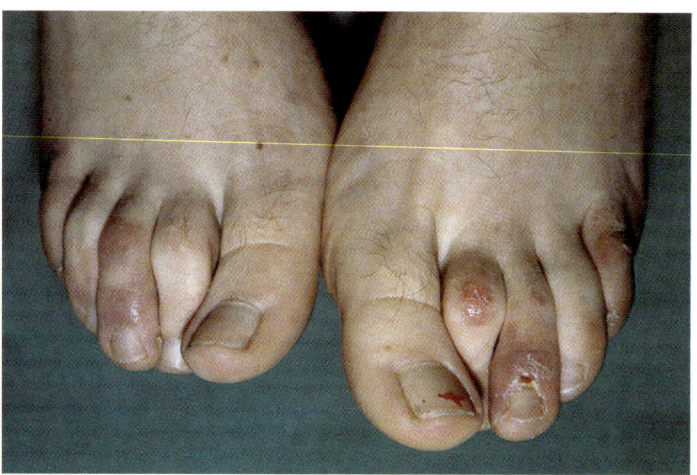

Figure 5.38
Chronic perniosis. Chronic perniosis in young woman; 6 years of seasonal recurrence.

HENNA

Henna is a dye obtained from leaves of three plants: *Lawsonia alba*, *L. inermis* and *L. spinosa*. The first of these is the most commonly used. These plants live in hot, dry climates, particularly in north Africa and Asia from the Mediterranean Sea to Iran.

Henna has long been used as hair dye because it produces a pleasant copper-like pigmentation. It is sometimes used as dye for the skin, often mixed with indigo, to tint the hands and feet. This practice is common in Saudi Arabia and Yemen.

Henna is a safe dye and cases of allergic contact dermatitis are rare. Henna should not be considered a true tattoo: the pigmentary effect persists for 3 months only.

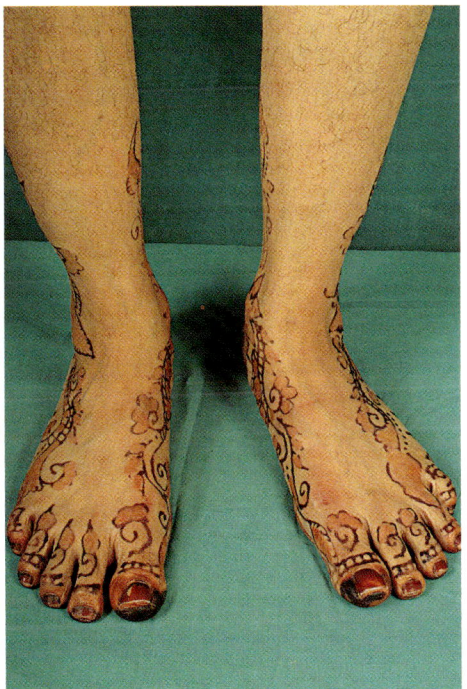

(a)

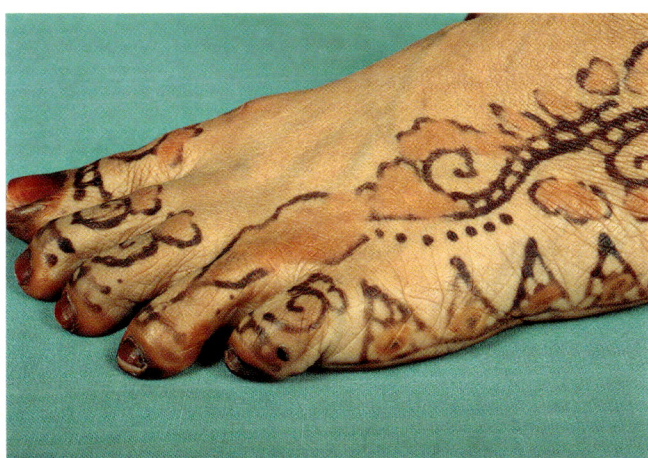

(b)

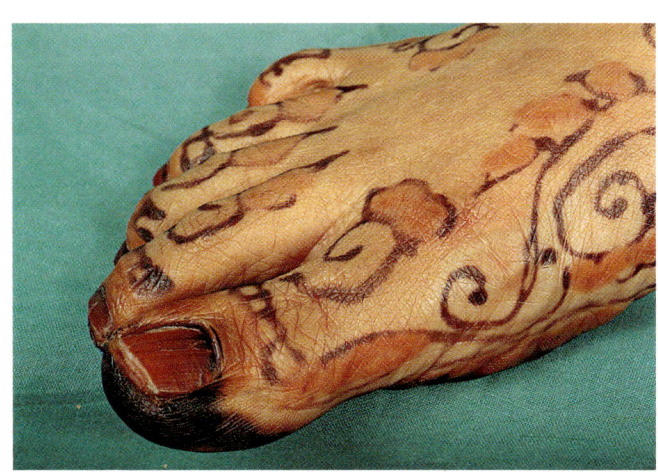

(c)

Figures 5.39(a–c)

Henna. The 'art' on the feet of an Italian woman returning from a trip to Yemen.

Index